The Gift of the Night

"No one can officiate a marriage between mind and spirit better than Philip Carr-Gomm."

~ **Ruby Wax,** actress and author of *Sane New World*
and *A Mindfulness Guide for the Frazzled*

"A brilliant, important, and inspiring book that will be so helpful to so many people."

~ **Rosalind Watts, Ph.D.,** clinical psychologist and clinical lead
for Imperial College London's psilocybin trial

"Sleep is one of the great unsolved mysteries of neuroscience. We understand very little of either what it is or why we, or indeed almost every animal that has a central nervous system, do it. With so little hard science as to its nature, those of us who suffer from sleep disturbances must fall back on empirical methodologies that have been shown to work. Philip Carr-Gomm's book is a practical guide to finding the peace that comes from returning to the patterns of sleep that energize our waking lives. I strongly commend it to you as a very practical and helpful guide."

~ **Peter Mobbs,** professor emeritus and former dean of
the faculty of life sciences and dean of preclinical
medicine at University College London

"Philip Carr-Gomm's message on how to access the power of the night for the world of healing, restorative sleeps, and dreams is of value and much needed. His six-step program provides practical and easy ways to fall asleep and to access your creative, healing dreams—an invaluable resource. I highly recommend *The Gift of the Night*!"

~ **Machiel Klerk,** author of *Dream Guidance*

"Sleep as a daily embodied spiritual practice! This workbook is a rare marriage of science and soul."

~ **David Peters,** professor emeritus and cofounder and director of the Centre for Resilience at the University of Westminster

"Philip Carr-Gomm presents a succinct but authoritative look at ways to help us sleep better. Science and spirituality are drawn upon equally, with inspiration and techniques coming via sophrology, yoga nidra, and the latest sleep research. The author even taps into the potential of psychedelic-assisted therapy, applying elements of the model as a way of optimizing the conditions for sleep. Accessible, practical, and endlessly thought-provoking, reading *The Gift of the Night* certainly won't send you to sleep, but the rich content contained within should provide even the greatest insomniacs with plenty of new ways to finally drift off."

~ **Ian Roullier,** cofounder of the Psychedelic Participant Advocacy Network (PsyPAN) and mental health advocate

"Philip Carr-Gomm has drawn on his own sleeping difficulties to create an integrative approach to tackling sleep issues. Although the problem is a simple one—we have difficulty sleeping well—the roots of it can be complex and multilayered. Philip draws on his training as a psychologist to help tackle these issues, combining the best of current scientific understanding with transpersonal approaches that help address wider holistic aspects of sleep disorder. Philip is highly trained in multiple disciplines (many of which contribute to the wide range of helpful suggestions in this book), but he wears his learning lightly. The book is written in a relaxed and conversational style: readers will feel as though they are being taken by the hand by a wise and helpful friend who can guide them toward a satisfying night's sleep. I can't recommend this book highly enough."

~ **Martin Treacy,** chartered psychologist and cofounder of the British Psychological Society Transpersonal Section

The Gift
of the
Night

A Six-Step Program for Better Sleep

Philip Carr-Gomm

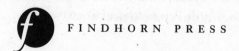

FINDHORN PRESS

Findhorn Press
One Park Street
Rochester, Vermont 05767
www.findhornpress.com

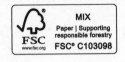

Findhorn Press is a division of Inner Traditions International

Disclaimer
The information in this book is given in good faith and intended for information
only. Neither author nor publisher can be held liable by any person for any loss
or damage whatsoever which may arise from the use of this book or any of the
information therein.

Cataloging-in-Publication data for this title is available from the Library of Congress

ISBN 978-1-64411-929-7 (print)
ISBN 978-1-64411-930-3 (ebook)

Printed and bound in the United States by Lake Book Manufacturing, LLC

10 9 8 7 6 5 4 3 2 1

Edited by Nicky Leach
Photos (p. 79) © Tina Stümpfig; Illustration (p. 79) © Mira Stümpfig;
with kind permission of Schirner Verlag, Germany
Text design and layout by Anna-Kristina Larsson
This book was typeset in Garamond and Halis R

To send correspondence to the author of this book, mail a first-class letter
to the author c/o Inner Traditions • Bear & Company, One Park Street,
Rochester, VT 05767, USA and we will forward the communication,
or contact the author directly at **www.philipcarr-gomm.com**.

Contents

PART TWO

Almost Everything You've Ever Wanted to Know about Sleep

Foreword

The power to intentionally alter consciousness is one of humanity's most important attributes. It is our mind's innate flexibility that permits us to imagine fresh perspectives, process emotions, restore our bodies, learn and solve problems, and have transcendent experiences. One state that embodies these properties exceptionally well is none other than what we instinctively do every night: We sleep and dream.

In previous eras, insomnia did not exist as the epidemic it is today. But sleep in modern culture has been impacted by more than just the introduction of artificial light. We live in a go-go-go, do-do-do, fast-paced society that is increasingly disconnected from nature. Not everyone is born with a temperament that can simply turn off their systems for responding to chronic stress in order to easily sleep through the night. Even if you're someone who doesn't feel your insomnia is explained by "stress", remember that stressors can be unconscious, too. These likely include some of the patterns you've developed to cope with insomnia in the first place that, paradoxically, contribute to maintaining it.

Fortunately, insomnia is reversible, especially with proven interventions like Cognitive Behavioural Therapy for insomnia (CBT-I). CBT-I teaches how to leverage the science of sleep, amend sleep-interfering beliefs and behaviours, and down-regulate the daytime stress and hyperarousal that impinge on quality rest.

As a psychologist who is board-certified in behavioural sleep medicine, I have witnessed the profound benefits of CBT-I, but I'm also aware of its limitations. Outcomes become even more compromised when insomnia is accompanied by common health troubles, such as dependence on sleep drugs or other substance use, chronic pain, menopause, mental afflictions, relationship problems, existential anguish, and the like. Moreover, some forms of CBT-I are taught with a cookie-cutter approach, requiring you to rigidly follow challenging instructions that restrict your time in bed to a shortened window. Limiting opportunities to be awake in bed deconditions your nervous system's associations between the nighttime environment and states of wakefulness while increasing your biological drive or "pressure" to sleep more efficiently.

Called sleep restriction and stimulus control, these therapies, which are based on learning principles as simple as Pavlov's dog or a rat in a Skinner box, can quickly rewire your brain to surrender to a peaceful, consolidated slumber. Unfortunately, some find these hard to commit to, usually because they require at least a few days of increased sleep deprivation to work. Even if you modify this approach to be less restrictive, or you diligently follow these and other CBT-I steps, your insomnia may not completely resolve.

Does this mean you have to resign yourself to a life of insufficient sleep, or say, using sleep medications? My belief is no. What I have found is missing from conventional therapies is something you will find in this book: The mind-body-spirit connection between sleep and the human penchant for altering consciousness. Herein, Philip Carr-Gomm weaves select, science-backed advice with vehicles of consciousness exploration, touching on areas including psychedelic medicine, meditation and yoga nidra, self-hypnosis, sound therapies, dreamwork, and lucid dreaming. Not only do such tools have hypnotic and trance-inducing features that can teach you to downshift into sleep, they also have the potential to introduce you to new, soul-nourishing possibilities.

One tool I believe some of the insomnia-prone have a hidden talent for is lucid dreaming—a state of explicitly knowing you're dreaming that enhances access to valuable experiences, resolving inner conflicts, and a deep, creative intelligence. Why? For one, the odds of lucid dreaming are known to increase when you infuse more wakefulness and vigilance into the night, something with which insomnia sufferers are familiar. Secondly, people with insomnia often experience *sleep state misperception*—a state of believing you are awake when you are objectively asleep. This hypervigilance during sleep can be reshaped to lend a type of awareness that not only eases wake-to-sleep transitions but also helps you to lucid dream. With the right mindset, your insomnia propensity could be an advantage in discovering how the borders between what is considered "awake" and "asleep" are not as rigid as you might think.

All told, the integrative perspectives highlighted in this book, combined with its practical suggestions, may be just what is needed to transcend your restlessness. Of the many books on this topic, I believe Philip's voice will guide you in finding that your insomnia is not an unsolvable mystery. Rather, it could be one of your greatest teachers in learning about higher-order consciousness and how to strengthen the intuition that bridges waking, sleeping, and dreaming.

Kristen LaMarca, Ph.D., DBSM
Clinical Psychologist, Diplomate in Behavioral Sleep Medicine,
certified by Board of Behavioral Sleep Medicine (BBSM)

Introduction

The Integrative Approach

LONG ago I learned how to sleep,
In an old apple orchard where the wind swept by counting
its money and throwing it away,
In a wind-gaunt orchard where the limbs forked out
and listened or never listened at all,
In a passel of trees where the branches trapped the wind
into whistling, "Who, who are you?"
I slept with my head in an elbow on a summer afternoon
and there I took a sleep lesson.

–From "Wind Song" by Carl Sandburg

Until a few years back, I never had any difficulty sleeping, so when my wife began suffering from insomnia, I didn't fully appreciate how devastating this could be. But then the gods decided I should learn what it felt like, and I went through a period of tossing and turning every night, either taking forever to get to sleep or waking in the middle of the night, only to find I couldn't drop back into sleep again. Lying awake, I was now caught in a loop of worrying that I wasn't asleep and then worrying about the fact that I was worrying.

My journey into the world of sleep research and therapy began in earnest, and here I am today, sleeping well again and teaching a system I've developed to help others sleep well, too. In a nutshell, it combines what we know about how to sleep better from scientific evidence-based approaches with methods that may not have any research evidence to support them but which many people find highly effective.

If you've experienced insomnia, you'll know how truly awful and debilitating it can be. This book is dedicated to making sure you never have to experience it again.

We all need sleep. Every animal, down to the tiniest flea, needs it. We're not entirely sure why our bodies need to sleep regularly—scientists can't agree on its main function—but we know we need it to stay alive. So if sleep is so essential, why is it sometimes so elusive?

If you are having trouble sleeping, welcome to the club. Some studies suggest that a third of the adult population has difficulty sleeping, and now poor sleep is becoming more prevalent due to the stress and altered lifestyles caused by the pandemic.[1] This phenomenon even has a name for it now: "coronasomnia".[2] It's getting worse for children and adolescents, too, thanks to social media, smartphones, and tablets.[3]

It may offer some small comfort to know that you are not alone with this problem, but what you really want to know is: "How can I change this and get a good night's sleep—every night?"

There are two approaches you can take in trying to solve your problem: the mainstream, evidence-based approach to insomnia recommended by doctors, or the alternative route, using methods like hypnosis or yoga nidra, which your doctor is unlikely to recommend because there haven't been enough double-blind trials to prove they work, even though many people swear by them.

In this book we take an integrative approach. The neuroscience and psychology of sleep is now well developed, and it makes sense to use techniques that have been scientifically proven to work. But it also makes sense to use methods that thousands of people have found effective over the years, too—even though the clinical research hasn't yet been undertaken to conclusively prove their value. Trying both of these approaches is a good idea because we are all so different. There is no one-size-fits-all when it comes to tackling insomnia.

See it like cooking. In this book, I'm going to present you with a whole bunch of ingredients and recipes that you can try out to find which ones work best for you. But more than that, I'm going to show you how to combine both approaches—the "scientific" and the "alternative"—so you'll have a greater chance of success with improving the quality of your sleep.

I'll do this by suggesting a Six-Step Program that puts together everything presented in this book in a sequence that's easy to follow. Because one size doesn't fit all, please feel free not to follow the program and to just pick and choose the methods you feel like trying.

But I recommend trying out the program first. Over the years, through my online sleep clinic and face-to-face with individuals, I've found it has helped so many people, and it offers you a discipline—a clear path forward—that can really help when you are suffering from the stress of not sleeping well. Just one idea in this book might be enough to help you sleep better.

Seasoned sleep therapist Dr. David Lee recounts cases in which just one suggestion solved his patients' problems.[4]

For example, as people get older, the muscles controlling their bladder get weaker and they find themselves waking often during the night to visit the bathroom. If each time you wake up, you find it hard to get back to sleep this can be annoying, if not debilitating. Lee talks to his patients about the circadian rhythm, and the way in which every 90 minutes or so they are going to be sleeping very lightly and can easily be awoken. Then he asks them to reduce their fluid intake prior to bedtime, gradually pushing back the time a drink is taken until they find their problem diminishes or disappears. It sounds almost absurdly simple or obvious, but sometimes we need simple advice.

Students of my online sleep course also sometimes report that just one technique fixes their problem. It might be one of the techniques given in Step 5—most frequently the Autogenic scan or the Sophrology exercise. Or it might be just one audio recording that hits the spot.

For example, one Amazon reviewer reported that my Healing Sleep audio track has successfully sent her to sleep more than 800 times. But for a lot of people, just one technique, one sleep "hack", isn't enough. And this is where a program like this comes in. For many people, improving the quality of their sleep is a more gradual process, with improvements coming slowly, perhaps with setbacks now and again, but the main thing is not to worry. Whether your road to better sleep is short and quick, or longer with some ups and downs, the research proves that insomnia can often be cured.

Cognitive Behavioural Therapy for Insomnia (CBT-I), the most recommended approach by the medical community because it is evidence-based, is proven to work for 70 percent of patients.[5] It uses a combination of education, encouragement to think differently, methods of relaxation, and the development of a good routine. You will find these same components in the approach advocated in this book.

Only two methods advocated in CBT-I are not included here. One method insists you never spend more than 10–15 minutes in bed if you are not asleep. The other method, called "sleep restriction", limits the total time you allow yourself in bed. Both methods are tough to follow, and you need to enrol in CBT-I therapy to make them work. The approach we take in this program is different and gives you different techniques to try. It lets you stay in bed, even if you're not sleeping.

CBT-I was born out of Behavioural Psychology, which engages with us as creatures susceptible to conditioning. The father of this approach was the Russian psychologist Ivan Pavlov, who experimented with conditioning dogs by using their salivation response. While we are all subject to conditioning, and working with this in a positive way is clearly effective, the approach we are taking in this book comes from a different perspective. Born out of Transpersonal or Spiritual Psychology, it suggests that in addition to us being animals that can be conditioned to change our behaviour, we are also spiritual beings whose souls need feeding, too, and who are the ultimate source of agency in our lives.

So the approach in the Six-Step Program offered in this book is to use most, but not all, of the methods that CBT-I uses, since they have been proven to be effective, and then to add in methods that speak to our souls, too.

* * *

Before we dive in, a word of warning (or I hope, relief). There are plenty of books about the physiology and psychology of sleep and about sleep research and the history of this research.

It's all fascinating stuff, but this book isn't going to tackle any of these subjects in depth. That's because the books have already been written, and the main purpose of this book is to get you sleeping better as quickly as possible.

Specific information about the science of sleep, which has been found to be therapeutically effective for those wanting to tackle their sleep problems, and which often forms the basis of the first one or two sessions of CBT-I, is included in Part One of this book. In Part Two, you'll find a lot of practical information about how to tackle specific problems and how to get the best out of your night's sleep.

If you find you are interested in the topic of sleep in general and want more information, do pursue this, because harnessing your curiosity is one of the best ways to reframe a problem in a positive way. Research has shown that bibliotherapy or psychoeducation—in other words, therapy from reading books and now, watching videos—does seem to help people sleep better. Although no one is quite sure why, the likelihood is that this is because, in learning about the topic, you develop a sense of control or agency, rather than feeling a passive victim of the problem. You'll find lots of resources to help you do this at the end of this book.

PART ONE

The Six-Step Program to Get You Sleeping Better

☾

Step 1

What Psychedelic Therapy Can Teach Us

*Here you learn how to start thinking and feeling differently
about sleep and the night itself, in ways that create the
foundations for sleeping better.*

There is a model being used today in psychedelic therapy that I have found also works really well in the field of sleep therapy. I'd like to share it with you here, because it can provide an incredibly useful map for the path towards better, healthier sleep.

But what on earth is "psychedelic therapy"?

Probably the most exciting and cutting-edge research in neuroscience and mental health today involves the use of psychedelics. With changes in legislation in many countries, research projects in over 60 universities around the world, and vast amounts of funding pouring into the field, scientists are exploring the potential for psychedelics, such as psilocybin, ketamine, DMT, MDMA, and LSD, to effect dramatic breakthroughs in the treatment of a diverse range of conditions including anxiety, depression, and PTSD.

Back in the Sixties, two Harvard psychologists, Timothy Leary and Richard Alpert (who became the spiritual teacher Ram Dass), popularized the use of psychedelics to enhance human potential. They discovered that they could also radically improve the treatment outcomes for a variety of problems, including those which have traditionally

17

been hard to treat successfully: addiction, alcoholism, and recidivism. By 1970, any use of psychedelics, whether for research, recreational, or therapeutic use, was outlawed, and it is only in recent years that researchers and clinicians, and the psychiatric world in particular, have become interested again in the healing powers of these substances.

Leary and Alpert's extensive experimentation taught them the critical importance of two factors that were necessary to get right if their subjects were to have positive and healing, and often mystical, trips. They expressed these as "set and setting".

If you take these powerful substances, which can in certain instances trigger severe negative reactions, including psychosis, you need to take them in a warm, supportive setting: in the company of loving friends, or with a skilled professional, if taken in a therapeutic context; in an environment where you won't be disturbed, surrounded by beautiful objects, ideally close to nature, with soft lighting, the right kind of music, and so on. Not a club. Not on a city street or on a bus or train. Not with people you don't trust. That's the "setting" part.

But what does "set" mean? Coming from the term "mindset", this refers not to the outer situation, the logistics of where you intend to take a journey that can take hours to unfold, but to your internal situation: your emotional state and your state of mind, your attitude, your approach to the quest you are about to undertake. If you are feeling confused, unbalanced, insecure or fearful, this is likely to negatively impact your experience.

In addition to set and setting, there is one other rather obvious factor that will influence your trip: the trigger, the drug itself, its nature, and dosage.

In essence, psychedelic journeys are experiences in consciousness. We shift from our everyday awareness to a decidedly different state of consciousness. In sleep, we do the same thing. If you suffer from insomnia, you are suffering from a difficulty in making that shift—from the waking state to that of sleeping and dreaming. For this reason, the understanding of the power of set and setting used in psychedelic therapy for making successful journeys into altered states translates very well into use for sleep

therapy, and it will guide our journey through the six steps I am now going to outline for you.

First, we'll work on "set": getting our internal state right—of our hearts and minds in Steps 1 and 2, and our bodies in Step 3. Then, in Step 4, we'll move on to "setting". In all this, we'll be attending to those things that come under the category of "sleep hygiene", an awful term used by doctors, which suggests that before we knew this stuff our sleep was unhygienic, somehow grubby. How rude!

Once we've got set and setting sorted, in Step 5, it's time to choose the method that will help us get to sleep, our equivalent to choosing the drug and its dosage in psychedelic therapy. Here, I'll offer you 13 ways to get to sleep.

Finally, in Step 6, we'll bed this all down for the long haul by building a morning and evening routine that fosters the best possible pattern of sleeping for us.

Let's begin by setting the stage and asking a big-picture question: What exactly are we dealing with here when we tackle the subject of sleep?

Quite simply, a third of our lives: its quality and how we relate to it. Since we spend this third of our lives asleep—or trying to get to sleep—it's worth our attention to get it right. It's foundational. If we can experience this time as being really helpful and inspiring to us, then we're well on the way to improving and working on the other two-thirds of our lives that we experience when fully awake.

Some people think that the time we spend in bed is wasted because we are not conscious. That's why they get into sleep hacking, trying to sleep less so they can be more productive. But they're really missing the point and falling into the trap, the hubris, of the ego, the rational conscious self that thinks they're the only kid on the block. The whole point is that this third of your life is not lost; it isn't even a time of blankness or unconsciousness, when nothing is going on.

In reality, it's a time when another part of you is able to soar, to breathe freely and experience life in a different way. It may be dark or inaccessible to your conscious mind, but your unconscious, your soul, your deep self, is alive and well during this third of your life. It makes sense to honour this and see how these two parts of yourself—your conscious and unconscious minds, your ego and your deep self—can cooperate to give you the fullest possible experience of life.

When you drift into sleep, you are not dropping into nothing-ness; you are dropping into another world that is rich in potential for healing, for problem solving, for creativity, for inspiration and for spiritual development. This book suggests ways in which you can work with all of this. It's focused on improving sleep quality and how to fix the problem of not being able to get to sleep or stay asleep easily, but all the while it's engaging with this other subject too, of discovering a rich inner life.

During the time you sleep, magic happens: an extraordinary sequence of events that is designed to change your consciousness, to free you from the ties of the everyday mind. Sleep pressure that has been building through the day, encouraged by the release of the hormone melatonin, and most likely coinciding with a trough in your circadian rhythm, tips you into the first stage of sleep. Your muscles twitch, your limbs might jerk a little, and whatever images you might be seeing become surreal as your everyday self loses its grip and you drop into another world, where the normal rules of life on the surface just don't apply.

Sleep pressure comes from the gradual accumulation of the neuro-transmitter adenosine within the brain. The levels of melatonin, a hormone produced mainly by the pineal gland in the brain in response to darkness, begin to rise about two hours before you go to bed. With adenosine and melatonin at work on your behalf, all you need to do is cooperate.

Your circadian rhythm will be helping, too. This regular rhythm of around 90 minutes continues day and night, affecting a host of func-tions, including hunger and thirst, urine production, alertness, and even creativity. During the day, you might only notice the rhythm when you hit that afternoon dip in energy, but in reality it's always there, cycling you up and down the hill of alertness. When you reach a low point of the rhythm in the evening, and it meets the wave of sleep pressure, that's the time to go to bed. But the rhythm will continue, taking you through five or six complete cycles each night, consisting of phases of light and deep sleep and the mysterious Rapid Eye Movement (REM) sleep.

You spend about half your sleeping life in light sleep, in various periods throughout the night. Your heart rate and breathing decreases, your brain activity slows down, but during this time little spurts of electrical activity occur, which scientists believe indicates your brain is transferring information from short- to long-term memory. This is why light sleep after study helps you retain information.

In deep sleep, your brain waves slow down; your metabolism of glucose increases, which helps memory consolidation and learning; your immune system is strengthened; and as the pituitary gland releases growth hormone, your body regenerates cells and repairs muscle and tissues. This restorative slow-wave sleep takes up 15–25 percent of your night's sleep time, about 1 to 2 hours in total.

As you get older, you tend to experience less of this deep sleep, but it's during deep sleep that an extraordinary process occurs. Up to 60 percent more space is created between the neurons that make up the brain in order to allow your cerebrospinal fluid to wash through it and flush out the build-up of a protein called beta-amyloid, which can form a sticky plaque that eventually kills brain cells and is found in Alzheimer's disease.

While all this is happening, you are in no way comatose. "Nothing could be further from the truth," says neuroscientist and founder of the Center for Human Sleep Science, Matthew Walker, in his book *Why We Sleep*.

What you are actually experiencing during deep NREM [Non-REM] sleep is one of the most epic displays of neural collaboration we know of. Through an astonishing act of self-organization, many thousands of brain cells have all decided to unite and 'sing', or fire, in time . . . Their voices have joined in a lock-step, mantra-like chant—the chant of deep NREM sleep . . . In this shamanistic state of deep NREM sleep can be found a veritable treasure trove of mental and physical benefits for your brain and body.[1]

When you're not in light or deep sleep, you're in REM sleep. It's during this time that most of your dreaming occurs, though you can dream in the other stages, too. Your breathing becomes irregular, and your heart rate and brain wave activity increase, while your body secretes two kinds of chemical to prevent your muscles moving. The partial paralysis, or loss of muscle tone, this causes is triggered to prevent you acting out your dreams.

You reach your first bout of REM sleep about 75 minutes into your first cycle, and then with each subsequent cycle the time spent in REM sleep extends a little, which is why you experience more time dreaming in the morning before you wake up. The total time spent dreaming adds up to about two hours each night, though you remember only a fraction of this time on awakening. REM sleep is important for your psychological health, your emotional regulation.

The overall picture of these three sleep phases, which recur in five or six cycles each night of around 90 minutes each, makes up what is known as your "sleep architecture", a pattern that is changed by sleeping pills, alcohol, marijuana and psychedelics, amongst other things, and which changes naturally too as we age.

Throughout the night, the duration of each phase changes, and in each of them, different things are happening: memories are being laid down; cells are being regenerated; dreams are being experienced; and the unconscious is speaking to us, resolving emotional conflicts and coming up with solutions to problems and attempting to release emotional tensions that have built up in reaction to events that have occurred in the previous days. And when dreams bring inspiration, messages from loved ones who have gone before us, premonitions of what may occur to us or others, or experiences of divine union or transcendence, then perhaps we are glimpsing the life of the soul within us.

The big takeaway from this book, and this approach, is that the night and sleep are not to be feared or resented; instead, they are to be welcomed as gateways into an experience of the life of the soul, of the unconscious, that offer the potential for a form of embodied spiritual practice. This has the additional advantage of bringing physical benefits as we learn how to sleep better.

The Gift of the Night

Let's get going with Step 1! Some people find it helpful if they can label their problem, while for others this is of no use or interest.

In case you're in the first category, let's define the issue this program addresses: insomnia. Doctors recognize two kinds of insomnia: acute (or temporary), if it lasts less than three months, and chronic (or long-term), if it lasts longer. Within these two categories of acute and chronic, the problem can manifest either as a difficulty in falling asleep at the beginning of the night, known as "sleep onset insomnia", or waking up in the middle of the night and finding it hard to get back to sleep, known as "sleep maintenance insomnia". If you're unlucky, you can suffer from "mixed insomnia", having both kinds simultaneously.

While most people suffering from insomnia can be helped with the various approaches discussed in this book, it's important to know that there are certain medical conditions that can be associated with poor sleep, and that these conditions need addressing with your doctor, regardless of whether or not your sleep improves by following the suggestions in this book. These conditions include sleep apnea, heart disease, hypertension, asthma, certain allergies, Parkinson's disease, restless legs syndrome, chronic pain, hyperthyroidism, attention deficit disorder, depression, bipolar depression, narcolepsy, and psychosis.

In general terms, a healthy lifestyle, sufficient exercise, a good but moderate diet, and plenty of sunlight and fresh air are all going to help provide the best conditions for you to avoid insomnia and sleep well. However, there are three negative factors that require attention when it comes to ensuring the optimal conditions for good sleep. Their prevalence may well be responsible for much of the contemporary pandemic of insomnia: reduced connection and contact with the natural world, stress engendered by our modern lifestyle and work patterns, and conflicts that may be occurring for us at the emotional level. It's well worth having a look at how you score on these three issues.

Are you getting out in nature enough? Do you get enough daylight? Do you commune with the birds, bees, and trees sufficiently? All this helps you not only feel good but also puts your body back in touch with that all-important circadian rhythm, as well as the rhythm of the year and its seasons.

Then ask yourself how you are doing with your stress levels? Does your work or family life create levels of stress or anxiety you need to address? If this is the case, some kind of approach that reduces your stress should be pursued. The daily practice of mindfulness meditation, yoga, tai chi, or qi gong all help; sophrology is highly effective and specifically designed to reduce stress, and yoga nidra is an excellent resource too if you're feeling anxious or stressed (you can read about these last two methods later on in the book).

Finally, take a look at your emotional life. Is it reasonably good, or is conflict occurring here? If so, then that needs addressing as well, perhaps with a counsellor or therapist.

Attending to these three aspects of your life won't necessarily get you sleeping better straight away, but it will certainly contribute not only to your overall sense of wellbeing but also, in the long term, to your ability to sleep better consistently, and it will enhance the application of the six steps you are about to take.

Avoid Orthosomnia: Throw Away the App or Sleep Tracking Device

Right from the start, you need to ditch any app or wearable device that is supposed to track your sleep. Although designed to help people, sleep specialists now believe these devices are responsible for a growing problem: insomnia triggered by the micromanagement of sleep. They've even given it a name: orthosomnia.

Research published in the *Journal of Clinical Sleep Medicine* puts it clearly: "There are a growing number of patients who are seeking treatment for self-diagnosed sleep disturbances, such as insufficient sleep duration and insomnia due to periods of light or restless sleep observed on their sleep tracker data." [2]

These patients are usually unaware of the fact that our needs for sleep vary and that you do not need to comply with a norm. The data supplied by the app isn't that accurate, and simply creates the wrong mindset: It feeds the worrier inside us. If you aren't sleeping well, you will know it by how tired and unsatisfying your sleep feels.

You don't need an app to tell you this, and you certainly don't need information that will make you anxious and might result in the nocebo effect, whereby you actually develop insomnia because you are told you are experiencing it. Orthosomnia can be very easy to cure if you move your app to the trash, or throw your Fitbit away.

The Power of Reframing

Worry is the enemy of sleep, and you need to find a way to eliminate it. This is easier said than done, of course, and the last thing you want is to be so concerned about worry that you find yourself double-worrying: worrying about the fact that you are worrying because you know it is harmful.

Let's be honest and confront the elephant in the room here—only in this case, it's not an elephant, it's a dove. There's a problem with this book—a problem with every book, course, or treatment method designed to help you sleep better. It is summed up in the words of the Austrian psychiatrist Viktor Frankl: "Sleep is like a dove which has landed near one's hand and stays there as long as one does not pay any attention to it."

This book is full of suggestions about how you can encourage that dove to come and land on your hand. The risk is that you become so preoccupied, obsessed even, with sleep, that you worry about getting things right, so you end up trying too hard and risk scuppering the very project you want to succeed. You think about sleep and your lack of it too much and scare the bird away.

It's paradoxical: To overcome insomnia you need to make an effort and be prepared to do things differently, but you also need to relax into the process and not try too hard.

Frankl had a way of working with such a paradox. He encouraged his patients to try *not* to sleep, when all the time they had been trying to do the very opposite. You might like to give this a go by trying to stay awake as long as possible, with a book, music, story, or podcast playing. Whenever you feel sleepy, remind yourself you're trying to stay awake.[3] If this method works for you, you will build up sufficient "sleep pressure", as it's known, and you will fail magnificently in the task you set yourself. If it doesn't work, keep reading!

If you find that it's worry that's keeping you awake, you can try jotting down your worries in a journal beside your bed or on an app like WorryJournal, to clear your mind before you go to sleep. Some people find this works; others find it just gets them thinking, and can even be counterproductive (*Oh, my God, I didn't know my list was so long. And I've only just started!*).

I suggest another strategy, one that doesn't confront worry head-on but, instead, works at another level of the mind and heart. It involves using **the power of reframing** for the intellect and self-compassion for the emotional self.

Reframing simply means taking a different perspective on a particular topic, and has been shown to greatly enhance our ability to resolve a difficulty. As an example, if you treat a problem that you're facing as a challenge, rather than as an obstacle, not only are you more likely to solve the problem but you're also more likely to reduce the amount of stress and difficulty you have in actually working through the issue. Once you've grasped this, you can reframe the problem of not being able to sleep well as an adventure, a learning experience, a challenge.

Don't worry about trying to rationalize this. The interesting thing about reframing is that you can tell yourself that you're going to reframe the issue, look at it in a new way, without even having to give yourself reasons. You simply say to yourself, whenever you find yourself thinking in a negative or despairing way about the issue: *Ah, this is so interesting. This is a challenge that I'm going to face, and I'm going to succeed with this.* You harness your will, your curiosity, your determination, rather than feeling defeated at the very outset.

What is the challenge? As noted earlier, it will almost certainly be that you either find it hard to get to sleep at night or that you wake up after an initial round of sleep to find that you can't get back to sleep again, maybe for a very long time. Sometimes people experience both problems. Alternatively, it may be that you simply feel that you don't get a deep enough sleep. Or you may be experiencing all of these issues.

The first reframe is to treat your sleep problems as challenges that you are curious about and feel confident you will resolve. And here's another reframing thought you might like to try: Let go of thinking about how you need sleep, and instead, tell yourself that you just need rest. It's always frustrating and uncomfortable thinking about what you're not getting, whereas, as long as you lie down, you know you are getting rest.

And now here's another reframe that can be really helpful to take on board: Instead of being your enemy, the night can become your friend. If you dread having to face each night because you feel you won't get enough sleep and you'll have to battle through it, with this reframe you turn this around and see the night as offering a gift.

This may either seem like a small, insignificant idea or a step too far for you, but the idea behind reframing is to make use of the mind's power to shape your experience, and in that sense, your reality. The invitation here is to change the attitude from one that tends to use military terminology, such as "fighting the problem" and "battling through the night", into a way of approaching the issue that is friendly, warm, and expansive, rather than defensive, aggressive, or despairing. Rather than "beating yourself up" for your inability to sleep, try accepting the situation, being compassionate and kind towards yourself, and sensing instead the gift that may lie hidden here, as there is always some.

We shouldn't underestimate the power of such acceptance to help us in our reframing. An effective form of psychotherapy known as ACT (Acceptance & Commitment Therapy) combines the down-to-earth techniques of CBT (Cognitive Behavioural Therapy) with the spiritually informed approach of mindfulness meditation. It works with the following basic truth about the way the mind seems to work: that what we resist persists, and that paradoxically, we are more likely to be able to effect change once we allow ourselves to fully accept our experience as it is, rather than fighting it.

Taking Step 1 in this program involves **accepting all your feelings and thoughts** about your experience of the night; that is, not fighting or railing against them, but instead, simply accepting them and becoming open to the idea that every night may have a gift for you and you are going to make sleep your friend. In this way, you open up to all the possibilities the night can offer, particularly during those times when you're lying in bed but not sleeping.

How do you do this?

We are all faced with so many demands on us, so many stresses, it's common for us to complain that we have no "me time", no time to order our thoughts, or listen to music, or meditate, or just be still, on our own, giving ourselves time simply to be. But the reality is that we're given at least eight hours every night when we go to bed, and it's just us lying there with plenty of "me time".

If you approach the night as an opportunity for a mini-retreat, you can start to sense it, reframe it, as a gift of your own personal retreat time. And if you can't get to sleep during this time, try reframing the issue not as one of "Why am I not sleeping?" or "How do I get to sleep?" but "What shall I do with my consciousness as I lie in bed?"

As long as your body and mind can be refreshed during the night, and as long as you can wake up feeling rested, then the problem isn't really about whether or not you actually go to sleep, or for how long you sleep. **The problem, or question, is simply what are you going to do with your consciousness?**

This way of reframing your problem is not a coverup of the underlying issue: that a lack of sleep is affecting you; it's the first step in resolving your difficulty. Rather than worrying about the fact that you're not getting enough sleep, you are approaching the issue with curiosity and interest and a kind of open-hearted welcoming of the potential of the night. You begin by *not* focusing on trying to resolve the difficulty you have with sleep.

A comparable situation is the difficulty you might experience when trying to meditate: If you try too hard, it simply doesn't work. On the one hand, you have to perform this quite subtle act of having sufficient motivation, will-power, and discipline to actually do the meditation and stay with it, while, on the other, relaxing into it, not trying to get anywhere, not trying too hard, and somehow instead allowing the meditation to unfold.

It's exactly the same thing with insomnia and inviting sleep. You have to have the discipline to engage with the issue and resolve to sort it out but not do battle with it. The trick is not to try too hard—and certainly not to worry.

Neuroscience tells us that we build physical pathways in our brains as a result of what we habitually think, feel, and do. As you start thinking and feeling about sleep and the challenges you face differently, and actually start to do things differently—as you soon will in the steps that follow—you will be creating new neural pathways in your nervous system. It may take a while for these new pathways to take over in your consciousness, but eventually, they will be established and you'll find yourself sleeping better.

So that's why the first invitation is to make the shift from seeing yourself as having a problem to seeing yourself being faced with an invitation to an adventure. And that adventure is exploring your consciousness and using the gift of every night to dive into different levels of being. Some of these you will experience as wakefulness, some you will experience as dreams or being asleep, but you can tell yourself that you will experience all of these states as restorative, healing, and energizing.

If you're feeling sceptical about all of this, please just try; tell yourself that this is so, just for the moment. Do it as an experiment. Be a research scientist, be curious, and say: *Okay, just for the duration of reading this book and trying out its ideas, I'm going to tell myself that this is what I think.*

Changing our thinking isn't enough, though. We are emotional beings, too, and while reframing an issue can be tremendously helpful, if our hearts are still troubled, the reframing will be less effective.

Psychedelic research tells us that for the right "set", we need not only the right intentions—the most positive and helpful thoughts about what we want to achieve—but also to be feeling acceptance and trust and a sense of connection to the world around us.

If your ability to trust in life or other people is feeling undermined or hard to contact, then this may well be affecting your ability to sleep. If tensions or conflict in a relationship or in your daily life are present, it can be hard for your psyche to drop its guard and let go into sleep. It seems obvious, but not many books on how to sleep better suggest that you might actually need to address such trust issues in order to improve your sleep. Seeing a counsellor or psychotherapist may need to become part of your journey back to sleeping soundly.

Step 2

Tune In

*Here you learn about how your experience of
sleep is an important part of the story of your life.
You determine your sleep personality, your chronotype,
and work out the best time to go to bed.*

Some good news: Researchers have found that people consistently overestimate their lack of sleep, so you may mistakenly believe you are not sleeping as much as you really are.[1] You tell yourself, *I didn't sleep at all last night,* but even as you say this, you remember those dreams you had. Research suggests we "stitch together" our memories of the times we were awake, leaving out the periods of sleep we had in between, and hey presto, our memory tells us that we were awake endlessly!

Now that you've hopefully taken on board the need to reframe your approach to be ready to welcome the gift of the night, and to continue the work on creating the right set and setting for this, that little piece of information above shows us that it's worth taking some time to really think about our sleep life—to uncover its story.

I once gave a seminar on sleeping better to a group of managers of a chain of cafés in Brighton. As we sat around one evening in one of the branches after hours, sitting in a circle with glasses of wine, I invited each manager to share their experience of sleeping. One by one, they talked about the challenges and difficulties they faced getting to sleep or staying asleep. Some of them started off by saying they had no difficulties at all, but by the time they had heard their colleagues talking about their difficulties, they started to open up and be more honest.

Here are some of the things they said.

One young woman in her twenties, who started off by saying she didn't have any problems sleeping, admitted on the second round of sharing that she would curl up on a sofa and watch television until she fell asleep with the TV still on. Later, she talked about how it was because she was frightened to actually go to sleep. Others talked about how their partners' snoring kept them awake, which had led them to question whether they should start sleeping in separate rooms. Others suffered from sleep maintenance insomnia, also known as biphasic or dual-phased sleep, finding it quite easy to go to sleep but then waking up a few hours later, only to find that they were unable to get back to sleep easily, sometimes lying awake for hours before nodding off again.

What was interesting about this shared conversation that night in the café was seeing how everybody, even those who weren't experiencing sleep difficulties, still had a story to tell about periods when they hadn't slept well, and about what they had discovered about their sleep, or about themselves more generally.

It confirmed a basic tenet of psychotherapy: that talking about your life as a story is an extremely helpful way to understand yourself and begin to resolve any difficulties you're experiencing.

Creating a narrative has the effect of organizing the host of ideas and feelings you have about your life, which otherwise can seem chaotic or random. It has a way of organizing your sense of self so that you can see your life as meaningful, as going somewhere. It strengthens your sense of who you are and shifts you away from feeling victimized by a ceaseless flow of events and experiences to feeling more empowered and in charge of your life. In psychobabble it helps the shift from "outer-directedness" to "inner-directedness"; outer-directedness meaning leading a life believing that you're at the mercy of circumstance, and inner-directedness meaning leading a life where you feel you have agency in the world, the ability to direct your life.

Your sleep story is part of the wider story of your life, and you can explore and articulate it just to yourself or to a friend or therapist. This might be the time to share the journey this book will take you on with someone you know who also has trouble sleeping. If you don't know anyone who has this problem, ask around—you'll be amazed at how quickly you will find someone you know who has trouble sleeping, too.

Then you can do the following exercise together. If you're on your own, speak your response to the following questions into your voice memo. Write them down if you feel like it, or just think through or speak your responses out loud.

Here's the exercise: Try **telling your sleep story**. When did you first experience difficulties in sleeping? Was it related to any particular event? How long has it gone on for? How does it manifest? Does it change? Is it cyclical? Is it affected by the phases of the moon? Is it affected by your emotions? How would you characterize the difficulty you face? How would you describe it? And what are the effects on your body? What does your body have to say about it?

Your initial reaction may be that you know darned well what your sleep, and any lack of it, is like and how it makes you feel, but these questions are encouraging you to go into detail, to go a little deeper. At one level they are encouraging you to have a conversation with your body.

Continue by looking at your dream life. Do you remember your dreams? Do they go in seasons? Do you ever experience sleep talking or walking, sleep paralysis, frequent nightmares or "night terrors"? Do you trace the start of your sleep problems to the menopause or doing shift work?

Have you ever considered that you might have sleep apnea, which involves not breathing for sometimes numerous times during the night? If you or your partner notice that your breathing stops and starts while you sleep, or that you make gasping, snorting, or choking noises while you sleep; and you often feel very tired during the day, you need to check this out. Experts suggest that 1.5 million people in the UK are likely to suffer from sleep apnea, with only 20 percent having been diagnosed.[2] You can find an online test link in Resources. If you find you might have this condition, see your doctor right away.

It's important to note here that in telling your story, you're not looking for solutions or trying to fix anything. This is just a first step. You're scoping out the situation. Using the psychedelic therapy metaphor mentioned in the previous section, it's essential to get these first few steps of preparing the set and setting right; we'll get on to actual methods for helping you dive into sleep once we've set the scene and plumped the pillows.

If you go to a sleep clinic or see a specialist to work on your sleep difficulties, they will get you to fill out a long form where you rate yourself on a scale from 1 to 10 on many aspects of your sleeping and waking life. And then they might ask you to keep a "sleep diary" for a while to track your sleep patterns.

These are important and valuable tools that help the clinician understand the difficulties you're facing and what the best treatment program will be, but here we're working in a different way: on the value simply of articulating your story. There's nothing you need to do with this, except express it, so that it becomes, if you like, a picture or movie that you can see, rather than something that is only semi-conscious.

Just this work of bringing an understanding of your story into consciousness is valuable in itself, as anyone will know who has experienced good psychotherapy or even simply good listening and skilful questioning from a caring friend. It's not even about drawing any conclusions or finding any meaning in the story. A great deal of the value in this work arises out of simply doing it.

When giving his CBT-I trainings for the British Psychological Society, Dr. David Lee starts with an admonition to the psychologists listening: How many of them get their clients' sleep story? How many train in CBT-I so they can help their clients? Not enough.

Research shows that CBT-I is more effective than sleeping pills, yet why do most GPs in the UK prescribe the pills if a patient complains of insomnia? Mostly because they have no one to refer them to for sleep therapy, although in 2022, this pattern began changing, as online CBT-I was upgraded to the treatment of choice. Psychological and physical health depends on three pillars: diet, exercise, and sleep. While diet and exercise are well recognized and researched as vital to our health, sleep lags behind and needs more trained professionals who can deliver treatment.

When Should I Head for Bed?

Once you have a sense of the pattern and nature of your sleep life, you can look at a helpful way of coming to understand this pattern, which can also help you work out your optimal bedtime.

Begin by asking your body when it would like to go to bed each night. What does it say to you? Try asking this question without preempting the answer. Even though you think you know what the answer is, just try it. Sometimes people are quite surprised by their body instantly replying that they want to go to bed at a different time to the one usually picked. This may not be the case for you, of course, but see what sort of response comes up.

Now ask yourself if you're a lark or an owl. Do you feel better in the mornings or evenings? If you had to do a particular task that required concentration, would you pick the morning or the evening to do it? And depending upon your answer, ask yourself whether your bedtime matches this. If you're an owl and you feel best late at night, are you able to organize your life so you can go to bed late and wake up late, and vice versa?

Although we popularly talk about larks and owls in relation to our preferences for when we go to sleep and wake up, sleep specialists suggest there may be more than two chronotypes, to use the scientific term for our "sleep personality", our body's preferred time for sleeping.

US sleep specialist Dr. Michael Breus, for example, talks about four, rather than two, types of sleep personality, which he renames as Bear, Wolf, Lion, and Dolphin types. A quick online quiz he offers will tell you more and suggest which one you might be (see the link in Resources).

We don't necessarily stay with one chronotype throughout our lives. We might, when we're very young, be larks and wake up at the crack of dawn, wanting food. And then when we're teenagers, we may shift to being a different chronotype: We become owls and want to go to bed late and wake up late. And then the rest of our life, we might be, for instance, a bear in Breus's terminology, which he reckons represents about 55 percent of the population. Bears want to work between nine and five and go to bed around 10 and 11 in the evening.

I once had a client who complained of feeling wretched in the morning. He woke up depressed and found it hard to summon the motivation to get out of bed. He wanted psychotherapy to help him overcome this problem. We worked out his chronotype, and I suggested he change his lifestyle from trying to be a lark to being true to his type, the owl. Luckily, he was a freelancer and could do this without a problem. The effect was almost immediate.

Identifying your chronotype will help you get a sense of whether you should head for bed early or late, but to get more precise you need to determine your circadian rhythm. Do you experience an afternoon dip in energy? For a lot of people, it's between 3 and 4pm, and some of us like to take a nap then, but if you're attentive, you'll find these dips are occurring cyclically through your day, and night, too.

They're caused by your biological clock and the circadian rhythm it's responding to. An adult's circadian rhythm goes through one complete cycle every 90 or so minutes throughout the day and night. During the night, when you sleep, you go through these 90-minute cycles in a way that takes you through the stages of light and deep sleep, then dream sleep, before repeating again.

During the day, you don't notice these cycles so much, except perhaps at the afternoon dip, but try keeping a "yawn diary", just noting whenever you yawn, and you might well find that it's happening about every 90 minutes. What this means, is that every 45 minutes you'll either hit a peak or a trough in your energy, and this simple fact will allow you to calculate when it's best for you to go to sleep. Take a look at this diagram, which Dr. David Lee at Sleep

Unlimited believes offers the single most valuable piece of psycho-education when it comes to tackling sleep problems:

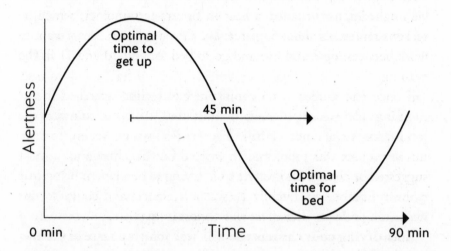

One cycle of the adult human circadian rhythm

This simple chart explains the phenomenon we've all experienced. You start feeling dead tired on the sofa. You realize you've got to get to bed. You turn off the TV, potter about in the kitchen, lock up the house, say goodnight to the dog, do your bathroom routine, and get undressed. Then you get into bed, and surprise surprise, you feel wide awake.

What's happened is that you've realized you need to sleep when your alertness is at its lowest, but by the time you've lain down, half an hour or so later, you're moving towards a peak of alertness in your rhythm.

To work out your own particular rhythm, just knowing one or two highs or lows should give you enough information. You tend to wake up naturally at a peak, so you then just calculate the 90-minute phases from then. Alternatively, you can use the time you feel your energy dipping as your starting point, or track your alertness over several days, noting when you yawn or feel particularly high or low in energy. Once you've worked this out, you'll know when it's a good time to head for bed and when there's no point. If at 10pm, you're at a peak, for example, don't expect to be able to go to sleep until about 10:45, so start the bedtime routine with enough time so that you're in bed by say 10:30pm. If you need reminding, set an alarm.

Note: The picture can be a little more complex, since we don't all have a circadian rhythm of exactly 90 minutes; that's just the average. The cycles can vary between 80 and 120 minutes, so bear this in mind when you calculate yours.

Once you've worked out the optimal time to start going to bed, this can help enormously in getting you off to sleep fairly quickly, but what if your problem is "sleep maintenance" and you find yourself waking up in the night, unable to get back to sleep?

This is very common, and there is a lot of evidence to suggest that this is a completely normal and natural phenomenon. It's called biphasic, dual, or segmented sleep, and researchers have uncovered historical evidence to suggest that sleeping in two segments with a period of wakefulness in between may well have been the way countless generations before us slept.

In his book *At Day's Close: Night in Times Past*, the historian Robert Ekirch cites abundant historical evidence that humans previously slept in two separated periods. He found more than 500 references to a segmented sleeping pattern in diaries, court records, medical books, and literature, from Homer's *Odyssey* to an anthropological account of modern tribes in Nigeria. Moreover, when researchers are taken down into caves or put into situations where they have no indications or knowledge of what time of day it is, with no exposure to natural light, they tend to sleep in two phases: the first for about two hours, followed by about four hours of being awake, and then in their second phase, they sleep for about four to six hours. So if you experience segmented sleep, you don't have to tell yourself you're suffering from insomnia. This is simply your sleep pattern.

Use auto-suggestion to tell yourself, *It's easy for me to fall back into sleep when I'm ready.* The emphasis is on *when you're ready*, because, of course, your experience has shown you that when you're not ready it's not easy. The auto-suggestion helps a positive framing of the issue, and when you are ready, if you need help drifting off, you can use one of the 13 methods suggested in Step 5. This then empowers you to do whatever you like during your wakeful phase, whether that means getting up, reading, using the gift of the night's retreat time for meditation or listening to music, and so on.

Once you've completed this second step in the program—coming to know your sleep story and working out your optimal bedtime—remind yourself of the key idea in the first step: trusting that the night holds a gift for you.

At the heart of this lies the belief that the issue is not about whether or not you're sleeping, but about whether or not you're getting rest and making use of this special time as a retreat, "me time", during which you can recharge and restore yourself. Every time you catch a negative thought about not being asleep, you flip it around and tell yourself that this is your time to do whatever you want to do with your consciousness: meditating, listening to podcasts, poetry, music. Lying down, just let those negative thoughts drift away . . .

And as you lie there, you might like to entertain the thought that you are actually already asleep, and that you might be experiencing "sleep state misperception": this is when you believe you are awake but are actually, by all objective criteria, fast asleep. In other words, your body is asleep, but you are experiencing a state of wakefulness, of self-awareness. When aroused from deep sleep, 5 percent of people report this experience, even though their body was by all measures soundly asleep.[3] Although this may sound unsettling, those with a spiritual orientation can find this inspiring. As your body rests, recharges, and repairs, your consciousness is free to meditate or try out some lucid dreaming! Sleep, and the time we spend preparing for it and slipping in and out of it, can become a daily embodied spiritual practice.

Step 3

Optimize the Body

*Here you learn about what you need to avoid, reduce,
or add to your diet or lifestyle in order to give your body
the best chance of getting a good night's sleep.*

In Steps 1 and 2, you have been working with developing the right "set" for your mind and heart: learning about sleep and your relationship with it, and perhaps changing your thinking and perspective around it (Reframing, or Cognitive Restructuring in CBT-I terms).

Now let's move on to consider the body. What can you do to set your body in order to optimize your chances for better sleep?

Certain illnesses will interfere with these chances, but CBT-I and sophrology are both used with cancer patients, for example, to good effect. Certain medications, such as beta-blockers and some anti-seizure and anti-malarial drugs, appetite suppressants, the decongestant pseudoephedrine, and thyroid hormone replacement drugs can also disrupt your sleep, as can the menopause, although hormone replacement therapy (HRT) is reported to alleviate this. Nevertheless, even with insomnia caused by these factors, the recommendations given in this program can be helpful. In particular, reframing sleeplessness in a positive light, as suggested in Step 1, can be extremely helpful when physiological factors make sleep hard to achieve.

First, let's look at what to exercise caution with and then move on to how you might fine-tune or optimize your body so that it's in the best state for sleeping well.

Sleeping Pills

When it comes to sleeping pills, the bottom line is that you want to try to avoid taking them for any length of time. If you're going through a crisis or a lot of stress and have been prescribed sleeping pills, don't be alarmed by the following information. Just try not to take them for too long. And make sure you consult your doctor if you want to stop taking them, so that they can ensure you do this in the safest way.

Neuroscientist Professor Matthew Walker, an expert on sleep, doesn't think taking sleeping pills is a good idea at all. Here are six reasons why, and to be clear, the following points refer to prescription medications like zolpidem (Ambien) and eszopiclone (Lunesta), not herbal pills or over-the-counter pills just using antihistamine, such as Nytol:

1   Sixty-five studies, involving almost 4,500 patients, found no difference in how soundly people slept whether they took a sleeping pill or a placebo. When you are given a sleeping pill you *do* go to sleep quicker, but you also go to sleep quicker if you *think* you have been given a sleeping pill! The team of leading doctors that researched this concluded that the effect of current sleeping medications was "rather small and of questionable clinical importance".

2   Despite the above, the drugs in these pills do affect your physiology. Pills such as zolpidem (Ambien) and eszopiclone (Lunesta) seem to produce sleep that is lacking in the largest, deepest brain waves when compared with naturally occurring sleep.

3   Side effects can include next-day grogginess, forgetfulness, and slowed reaction times in motor skills such as driving.

4   When individuals stop taking these pills, they may suffer from even worse sleep, which is known as "rebound insomnia". The brain has tried to alter its balance of receptors as a reaction to the drug. It has tried to "become somewhat less sensitive as a way of countering the foreign chemical within the brain", as

Prof. Walker puts it. This creates drug tolerance, and when the drug is stopped, as part of the withdrawal process there is a spike in insomnia severity. Rebound insomnia often results in patients reverting to taking the drug.

5   One of the functions of sleep is to "lay down" your memories; that is, to strengthen the neural connections between synapses that make up a memory circuit. That is why it is good to nap when you revise for an exam, rather than staying up all night "swotting". When you sleep, you are storing memories. Studies in animals given sleeping medication showed a 50 percent weakening (unwiring) of neural connections formed during learning. As Walker puts it: "Ambien-laced sleep became a memory eraser, rather than engraver." If it has this effect on humans (we do not know yet, but it seems likely), this is unfortunate for anyone taking these pills, particularly for those who are older, whose memories need strengthening not weakening, and for the increasingly younger population who are being prescribed the drug and need to learn in school or college.

6   Most worrying of all are the findings of Dr. Daniel Kripke, who has discovered that "individuals using sleep medications are significantly more likely to die and to develop cancer than those who do not." In 2012, Kripke compared 10,000 patients taking pills with 20,000 matched individuals not taking them. Those taking more than 132 pills per year were 5.3 times more likely to die. Even those taking just 18 pills a year were still 3.6 times more likely to die. Since Kripke's work, more than 15 other studies have been carried out with similar findings. The stats linking pill-taking with cancer are equally depressing: Within a two-and-a-half year period people who were taking pills were 30–40 percent more likely to develop cancer.

I have summarized these findings, but if you are concerned, do look at chapter 14 of Walker's book *Why We Sleep: The New Science of Sleep and Dreams*, listed in Resources, which goes into much greater detail and gives references to the research literature.[1]

So there you have six reasons not to take sleeping pills, or only very sparingly. But perhaps give a thought to how much you might be hurting the pharmaceutical industry if too many people deprive them of revenue. Walker gives a good comparison. One of the highest grossing movies of all time, *Star Wars*, took 40 years to amass $3 billion in revenue. The leading brand of sleeping pill, Ambien, amassed $4 billion in sales profits in two years. How come? In the USA alone, 10 million people will have taken a sleeping pill in the last month.

Amitriptyline

To avoid the problems of tolerance and addiction that can come with sleeping pills, some doctors prescribe the antidepressant amitriptyline to their patients. Used off-label for this purpose, amitriptyline's sedative effect can help induce sleep, and in such low doses the likelihood of potential side effects—such as dizziness, constipation, headache, and weight gain—are reduced. But because the drug remains active in your body for up to 24 hours, even at low doses you may well find yourself feeling groggy during the day and its impact on your psychomotor performance might mean it affects your ability to drive safely. In addition, it disturbs your sleep architecture, reducing the amount of deep sleep and REM sleep you are getting. The bottom line is that taking amitriptyline for a short period may help you fall asleep, but it is not addressing the root cause of your insomnia and risks interfering with the restorative processes that occur during deep sleep and dreaming.

Milk

Some people find a glass of milk or a warm milky drink taken just before bedtime makes them sleepy. Aside from the fact that drinking just before you go to sleep risks creating pressure in your bladder and the desire to urinate just when you want to be fast asleep, for many people digesting the fats in milk can keep them awake. Some people argue that the tryptophan in milk helps increase your melatonin levels, but you would have to drink two gallons for any noticeable increase to occur, and this would not take effect immediately anyway. Any positive effect on sleep from drinking warm milk is far more likely to be due to the fact that this has become a familiar part of a bedtime routine with associations forged between the drinking of warm milk then lying down to get ready for sleep, perhaps stretching back into childhood.

Alcohol

Having a drink before bed is the most common way that people self-medicate to help them get to sleep, but there's a problem here. Although alcohol does often make you sleepy, it reduces the amount of deep sleep you get, and over time this can become damaging, since it is during deep sleep that your immune system is strengthened, muscles and tissues are repaired, and the brain is flushed of toxins. If you drink, try to have two or more alcohol-free days a week, limit your intake to the daily recommended allowance, and avoid drinking at least two hours before going to bed.

Cannabis

Now that cannabis is legal in certain places, self-medicating with it for better sleep is on the rise. Companies are offering cannabis products designed specifically to induce sleep. For example, one company, Cresco in Illinois, offers a range that includes flowers, vapes, and concentrates. Edibles for sleep are popular, too. One product, Wyld's CBD Elderberry Sleep Gummies, CBD + CBN, has added sleep-inducing CBN (cannabinol) and is advertised as coming "in a 2:1 THC:CBN ratio with special indica terpenes to ensure the user falls asleep".

While many people find cannabis helps them sleep, some evidence suggests that it reduces the time spent in dream (REM) sleep and extends the time spent in deep sleep.[2] Dream sleep is needed for your emotional health, and any change to the natural architecture of your sleep—how long you spend in each phase—may not be in your best interests long term.

Cannabis for help with insomnia may be available to you legally in the UK via Drug Science's Project Twenty21. An alternative that is legal, and that avoids the psychoactive effects caused by the presence of any THC (Tetrahydrocannabinol), is CBD (cannabidiol, a compound extracted from the cannabis plant that has various benefits, but which unlike THC doesn't get you high). Research shows that many people buy CBD products in order to sleep better. Since CBD is said to reduce anxiety, it may be that a reduction in anxiety facilitates better sleep.

Nicotine

Nicotine is a sleep disruptor. It's a stimulant, which is why a few drags on a cigarette can perk you up if you're feeling sleepy. But in addition to smoking causing all sorts of health problems, it can exacerbate insomnia and increase your risk of developing sleep apnea. The trouble is, quitting can disrupt your sleep, too, as you suffer withdrawal symptoms and your body adjusts. Despite that, it's always worth giving up smoking!

Blue Light

Lots of people look at their televisions, computers, tablets, or smartphones in the evening, but these all emit short-wavelength-enriched light, known as "blue light", which interferes with your ability to sleep by disrupting the production of the sleep-inducing hormone melatonin produced mostly by the pineal gland. Even LED lighting produces blue light.

Some smartphones and tablets have "night-time viewing" settings that let you adjust the blue light emitted, and you can get a blue light filter for your TV and special blue light blocker glasses to wear, but sleep experts believe that it's not only the blue light that is messing with your sleep. Watching television and engaging with social media are highly stimulating activities compared with the sorts of things our ancestors would have done in the millennia before us.

If you find it hard to wind down and drift off when lying in bed, try winding down several hours before. Rather than dealing with email or watching the latest thriller, engage in relaxing activities such as reading, writing, listening to calming music, or taking a bath. If you do take a hot bath, you might find that taking it too close to bedtime means you are too hot and this stops you from getting to sleep, so make sure you take it earlier in the evening.

The bottom line is that you need just three things for a good night's sleep: a safe place to sleep that is cool, quiet, comfortable, and dark; a calm mind; and a relaxed body. Working out how to have a calm mind and body can be a challenge, but a good start is to look at those few hours before bedtime to see if you can create the optimal conditions for calm.

Toothpaste

If you stagger sleepily off the sofa to go to bed, only to find that the bathroom routine of brushing your teeth and so on actually wakes you up, do that an hour earlier, then, when fatigue hits, you can go straight to bed. It's also possible that if there's peppermint in your toothpaste it is acting as a stimulant, so switch toothpastes for the evening brush.[3]

Meal Times, Diet, and Sugar

You need to allow enough time for digestion before bedtime so that it does not interfere with your ability to get to sleep. As you get older, it's common to need more time between your evening meal and going to bed, so you might find that simply tweaking this detail in your life can make a big difference. You could try shifting your evening meal from say 8pm to 7pm or even 6pm, and see if that has an effect.

Some people, however, find that having a light bedtime snack or warm milky drink before going to bed can help them. But for most of us, eating in the evening gives us a boost of energy: the sugars in food are absorbed quickly by our stomachs and reach our bloodstream before any other nutrition. That's why you might find yourself snacking as you watch late night TV; your body really wants to go to bed, but you can eke a bit more out of your waking day by absorbing those sugars. That's why it's recommended, if you have any trouble getting to sleep, that you don't eat for at least two hours before you go to bed.

And again, just as so many issues are interrelated when it comes to our health and wellbeing, there will be foods that disturb your digestion and therefore disturb your sleep. Part of working on your wellbeing, and making sure that you sleep better, involves also making sure that you eat better.

Some people, for example, find that completely cutting out sugar helps them regulate their sleep. And some find that the Ayurvedic medical advice to avoid hot, spicy, or stimulating foods, such as chili, ginger, garlic, and onions, particularly in the evening, helps them sleep more easily. Herbalist and author Julian Barker gives his clients this advice: "Don't eat anything sweet before bed, except for yoghurt or ripe banana. The evening meal should contain some fat and protein with a complex carbohydrate such as rice."

Insomnia can also be caused by histamine intolerance, or excessive levels of histamine in the body. Histamine is a neurotransmitter that is involved in the body's immune response to injury, allergy, or infection. While we need a certain amount of histamine as part of our body's defences, if we produce too much this can cause a range of problems, including headaches, fatigue, skin complaints, and interference in our ability to sleep well.

Stress, an infection, post-viral syndrome, and environmental allergens can all provoke the overproduction of histamine. Antihistamine drugs are used to combat allergies, and a common side effect of these drugs is drowsiness, which is why certain over-the-counter sleeping pills like Nytol make use of antihistamine. Certain foods produce histamine, and by eliminating dietary histamine, some people report a dramatic improvement in the quality of their sleep. Taking activated charcoal about two hours after an early dinner is said to absorb excess histamine, and should only be used as a short-term measure in combination with a long-term approach following a low-histamine diet.

Caffeine

It's common knowledge that caffeine keeps you awake, so you need to avoid ingesting it after around 2pm. Remember that black tea also contains caffeine; it is not just found in coffee. Bear in mind that regular tea bags tend to give you more caffeine than loose-leaf tea, and the longer you brew it, the bigger the hit. You can lower the amount of caffeine you get from coffee by switching strengths. Different beans have different strengths: Robusta beans, for example, contain double the caffeine of Arabica beans. There is a growing list of coffee substitutes or real coffee with mushroom combinations that have less or no caffeine, and these can all help you reduce your daily caffeine intake. Simply switching to drinking decaffeinated coffee can also be effective. Research shows that even when we know it's decaffeinated, the placebo effect results in a reduction of withdrawal effects.[4]

Exercise

Research shows that people who don't take much exercise tend to have poorer sleep. Review how much exercise you take, and see if this needs increasing, even if only by a small amount. Research also shows that exercising too close to your bedtime can interfere with your sleep. It raises your heart rate, blood pressure, and body temperature, keeping you awake. So don't go out for a jog just before you plan to turn in! Exercise earlier in the afternoon or better yet, in the morning, and you will reap the rewards of this not only in sleeping better but also in an improvement in the quality of your life and your overall health. Some specialists recommend this simple rule of thumb for better sleep: Take regular moderate physical exercise for six days out of seven. If you are unable to exercise, simply sitting outside for 30 minutes a day can really help, as you will see in the next section.

Nature: the Great Healer

It's likely that the phenomenal increase in reports of insomnia is partly due to our modern urban lifestyle and its disconnection from the cycles and influences of the natural world. With artificial light, heating and air conditioning, and the time we spend in front of screens, it's no wonder. The more divorced we are from natural light and the life-giving powers of nature, the more our health is likely to suffer. When you spend a good deal of time outside and come back tired, people say it's the result of all that fresh air. It's not the air that's made you sleepy but your exposure to natural light.

One of the best things you can do for your overall physical and mental health as well as your sleep health is to make sure you spend time outdoors every day. Get back in touch with the seasons and the elements, the cycles of life, annual and diurnal. To encourage your body's production of melatonin and vitamin D, which are essential for good sleep, make sure you get at least 30 minutes of morning light on your skin, ideally direct sunlight, every single day.

Mushrooms

Traditional Chinese medicine has known for centuries that mushrooms can improve our health, and reishi (*Ganoderma lucidum*) mushrooms are often used to treat insomnia and chronic fatigue. Studies have shown that consuming reishi mushrooms can reduce the length of time it takes to get to sleep, as well as increase the amount and total duration of deep sleep.[5,6,7]

As with ingesting any substance, you need to be careful about reishi mushrooms, as they can have side effects. They are contraindicated if you take anticoagulant or blood pressure medications, and if used too regularly or in too great a quantity, they can actually cause insomnia. So it's best to take them infrequently and in low doses in consultation with a health professional. You can find reishi mushrooms offered in capsules, powders, and tinctures, but many people prefer drinking reishi as a tea.

Three other mushrooms are also said to help with sleep in a less direct and more supportive capacity: cordyceps (*Cordyceps Sinensis*), lion's mane (*Hericium erinaceus*), and chaga (*Inonotus obliquus*) mushrooms.

Enthusiasts claim that cordyceps can boost levels of cellular rejuvenation, stamina, and vigour, while lion's mane stimulates the growth of neurons (brain cells) and supports remyelination, which repairs and regenerates the sheathing of the axons, the nerve fibres that carry nerve impulses away from our cells. Chaga mushrooms, which grow in Siberia, Alaska, the northern US, and Canada, are known as "black gold" in Russia, and have been used traditionally to treat heart disease, diabetes, and gastrointestinal cancer, apparently by helping regulate the immune system and containing antiviral properties. Reishi are the only mushrooms to have been directly proven to have the potential to improve sleep; cordyceps, lion's mane, and chaga mushrooms appear to act in a more generalized way to regulate physical function, and thus, indirectly affect sleep quality. If you decide that you would like to take reishi mushrooms in conjunction with these other kinds of mushroom, it would be wise to consult carefully with an expert first.

Melatonin

Our sleep-wake cycle is to a great extent governed by the pineal gland in the brain, its secretion of the "sleep hormone" melatonin, and our experience of the circadian rhythm. Melatonin production peaks in the evening, and this signals to your body that it is time to go to sleep. Taking artificially produced melatonin can help you sleep, and is a favourite amongst some frequent flyers to combat jet lag.

Doctors do prescribe melatonin, it can be bought off-prescription in some countries too, but it should only be used in the short term. In the UK, doctors use it mainly with adults over 55, and ask you to stop taking it within four weeks, since there are risks of habituation and dependency. You need to avoid alcohol and smoking when taking it, and you may get an allergic reaction. Some people find it makes them tired, irritable, or nauseous, or it gives them a headache, and a number of ongoing health conditions, such as rheumatoid arthritis and liver or kidney disease, contraindicate it.

Since it shouldn't be taken long term and has so many caveats surrounding it, it is unwise to buy it off-prescription, and there is some evidence that the dosages normally suggested are far too high, and that melatonin works more effectively when microdosed. For more on this see page 129. In the final analysis, you are better off boosting your melatonin levels naturally by making sure you expose yourself to daylight, not light mediated through a window, and ideally sunlight, for at least 30 minutes—and preferably longer—every morning.[8]

Vitamins B, D, and Magnesium

Vitamin D and magnesium are two supplements worth investigating to improve your chances of sleeping well. Research shows that people with low levels of vitamin D tend to experience disturbed sleep patterns and shortened sleep times, and studies have shown improvements in sleep resulting from vitamin B and D supplementation.[9] There are other good reasons for taking these vitamins,, too, so as part of your preparation for sleeping better, consider taking them alongside magnesium.[10]

Research shows that magnesium can help people fall asleep quicker and sleep for longer.[11] It seems that taking magnesium can increase concentrations of melatonin, which leads to better sleep, and decrease cortisol, known as the "stress hormone". Magnesium supplements also seem to reduce the symptoms of what are known as "parasomnias", which are unwanted experiences that disturb sleep, such as sleepwalking, sleep paralysis, and "night terrors". In addition, certain enzymes in your body require magnesium to be able to convert vitamin D into its active form (known as calcitriol), which is why it's good to take them both.

Footbaths, Herbal Teas, and Other Supplements

Research shows that taking a warm footbath of around 40C (104F), 1–2 hours before bedtime, might increase the length of time you sleep.[12,13] While your feet are soaking, you could try a herbal tea such as chamomile or valerian, or a combination of the two; there are plenty of these on the market now. Valerian root supplements taken in tea or pill form as a sleep aid are popular in Europe, and increasingly in the US, and an analysis of 60 research studies has determined that, for many people, valerian has the effect of reducing anxiety, helping them fall asleep faster and experience improved sleep quality.[14, 15]

Ten minutes spent surfing online will show you all sorts of products that claim to help you sleep better. In addition to valerian supplements and herbal tea combinations, you can find the traditional remedy of a hop pillow; gummies with melatonin, California poppy, lemon balm, and cabbage rose; gummies with 5-HTP and passiflora; hops and saffron extract pills. Research is limited or nonexistent for most of these supplements, which is not to say they can't help. But for this reason, it might be wise to stick to the proven supplements— vitamins B and D, magnesium, and valerian—while avoiding the risks associated with melatonin.

Dialling back the time of your evening meal; going easy on the booze, coffee, and blue light; taking exercise; making sure you get natural light every day; perhaps taking proven supplements—these steps towards better sleep may or may not seem to make a difference, but trust in the science; they've all been shown to help. Give your body a chance to adapt, and know that you have now done all you can to fulfil the injunction to get your "set" right. Now you just need to attend to your "setting".

☾

Step 4

Prepare the Setting

Here, you learn how to create the best setting for your sleep, a sanctuary for drifting into the world of dreams, by paying attention to your bedroom and bedding; the qualities of light, sound, air, and temperature; with some unusual additions to the room that may be helpful and some attention to the problem of snoring.

In Steps 1 to 3 you worked on creating the optimal conditions for your body, heart, and mind. Now we're going to do the same thing for your outer circumstances. In psychedelic therapy terms, we're going to turn our attention from "set" to "setting". In that kind of therapy, you make sure the room and surroundings are beautiful and supportive for a journey into other realms of consciousness.

Going to sleep is an excursion into other levels of consciousness, too. Whether those other levels are personal and our dreams simply result from a dive into our unconscious, or whether something more extraordinary happens, is a matter of conjecture and belief.

Some thinkers, such as the famous teacher and clairvoyant Rudolf Steiner, would say it is a matter of inner knowing, too. Steiner believed that when we sleep our soul detaches itself from our physical body in order to journey into other worlds, which we see in our dreams:

In sleep the soul is independent of the life of the body, as a rider is independent of a horse . . . it has to withdraw from the body from time to time to draw strength from a region outside the body.[1]

The same idea can be found in Buddhism, with the Dalai Lama stating:

> Tibetan Buddhism considers sleep to be a form of nourishment, like food, that restores and refreshes the body. Another type of nourishment is *samadhi*, or meditative concentration. If one becomes advanced enough in the practice of meditative concentration, then this itself sustains or nourishes the body.[2]

The Dalai Lama goes on to say that advanced practitioners can create a "special dream body" from the mind and the vital energy of *prana*, or breath, in the physical body. This dream body "is able to disassociate entirely from the gross physical body and travel elsewhere".

Whether sleep represents a time when your dream body or soul leaves your physical body, or a time when your mind and heart can voyage in the depths of your own psyche, it makes sense that such an important activity should occur in a place of safety and beauty.

Churches, temples, and sacred sites are all places where you're invited to change your consciousness. They offer a gateway to the Otherworld. As liminal places, they invite you to step over the *limen*, the Latin word for "threshold", in order to enter another dimension of awareness. They understood this in the ancient world, and even built temples that were designed specifically for "sacred sleep" or "temple sleep", which the pilgrim would visit in the hopes of having a dream that would give healing or guidance.

Evidence for these temples has been found in Egypt and elsewhere in the Middle East, in Greece and Italy, and even in Britain. In 1928, an archaeology dig unearthed the remains of a Roman sleep temple at Lydney Park in Gloucestershire, and author J.R.R. Tolkien, in his role as a philologist, was called upon to investigate the Latin inscription there.

If you've ever had a dream that has had a healing effect on you—perhaps resolving some emotional conflict or reuniting you with someone you thought you'd lost—you'll know what is meant by a "healing dream". And of course, sleep in itself is healing, which is why it's such an important part of convalescence. We go to sleep in order to be healed, restored, and rejuvenated.

And where better to seek this restoration and these healing dreams than a place that is treated like a sacred place in itself, dedicated to the magical act of changing consciousness, voyaging in the Otherworld? If you think about it, it's pretty extraordinary that there is a dedicated room in your house or apartment devoted to this process of consciousness alteration. Rather than taking this for granted and not really thinking about it, if we take this idea on board, it enables us to approach our bedroom in a new light.

We're all familiar with the idea that "my body is my temple". In this new light, you might want to see your bedroom as your temple, too—a place where you let go of the awareness of your physical body in order for it to be recharged and regenerated; for your consciousness to voyage in the world of dreams, and perhaps of Spirit, too. Or you could see it as your sanctuary, or ashram: a place of peace and tranquillity. Imagine showing a friend around your new apartment: "And now, here's the room that is dedicated to changing consciousness," you might say as you open the bedroom door.

If you like this approach, then go into your bedroom now and ask yourself: "How can I organize this room to be an uplifting, inspiring place for the voyages of my soul?" Look at the colours that your bedroom is decorated in, the pictures that are hanging on the walls. Is it a room that acts more like a living room or storage space, or is it a place that really is dedicated to this sacred task of entering other realms?

Of course, there are constraints of space and time and money, and if you have a partner, whether they want to see the bedroom in the same way. But as far as you can, ask what you can do in terms of decluttering the room, decorating it in soothing colours, choosing just the right images to encourage your consciousness to transition to other levels.

There is some, admittedly slim, evidence that sleeping in alignment with the flow of the Earth's magnetic field, which runs North–South, will give you better sleep than if you are oriented against it, such as in an East–West direction; however, it's often not practical to reposition a bed, and be wary of consulting a feng shui guide to bed positioning, because if you can't move your bed much, it may introduce you to unhelpful and unproven ideas about why your bed is in the wrong place.

We know from science that a bedroom needs to be dark, quiet, well ventilated, and cool. So maybe you need to fit blackout blinds or thicker curtains, and if your night-time trips to the bathroom necessitate switching on lights, get one or more children's nightlights that plug in at floor level to guide you there, instead.

You might like to try using an eye pillow, which not only ensures you are not distracted by any light but also makes use of the oculocardiac reflex. This reflex, which comes from slight pressure on the eyes, has the effect of reducing your heart rate and blood pressure. It's possible, too, that the pressure stimulates the vagus nerve, which influences the heart, lungs, and digestive system, encouraging relaxation. You can get eye pillows that smell of lavender, which is said to encourage sleep, and you can warm or cool them beforehand, if you wish.

You might need to somehow make sure your bedroom is quieter, too, and that you've got a great mattress, a great pillow, and the bedding is just right. In very rare cases, some people get an allergic reaction to the detergents used for washing their pillow cases or bed linen, and this can interfere with their sleep.

You might want to play safe and eliminate your exposure to EMF (electromagnetic fields) from wi-fi and other electrical devices, which some people believe interferes with our sleep. Although the scientific consensus seems to be that no harm is likely to come from such low doses in domestic environments, it's simple to connect your router, and any other device near the bed, to a timer and program it to turn off at night. If you do this, you can also make sure your phone isn't by your bed, too.

Although experts say our bedrooms should be cool to aid our sleep, our bodies need to be warm, and some people report that wearing socks in bed helps to send them off to sleep. If your partner needs a different temperature to you in bed, consider getting two single duvets of different weights and putting them in a double duvet sleeve, so you both get the warmth you need. Some people find that sleeping under a weighted blanket helps them sleep better. It makes them feel more secure and safe, as if they're being hugged, and often say that it helps them with their anxiety as well as their insomnia. You can buy these online, with blankets adding from 4 to 25 pounds of weight. Be careful, though. There have been fatalities when such blankets have been used with babies or small children.

Breathing clean air helps you sleep better, too. Himalayan rock salt lamps are said to help with this, and NASA has carried out an interesting research project into plants that clean the air.[3] Here are the ones that they found do the job best: jasmine, lavender, snake plant, aloe vera, gardenia, spider plant, valerian, English ivy, peace lily, golden pothos, bamboo palm, gerbera daisies, and red-edged dracaena. You might like to have one or two of these potted plants growing in your bedroom.

Although there's no research to support this, it is often suggested that the smell of lavender promotes good sleep, so you could try a lavender pillow on the bed, or use essential oils or an aroma dispersing device that you can easily find online.

Animals and Snorers

As we consider the setting for your nightly trips into the Otherworld, we need to take into account whether you have a partner in your bedroom, human or animal, or perhaps both. If one or more animals sleep in the room with you, try not to be sentimental about this and really ask yourself whether this is helping or hindering your sleep.

It may well be that their companionship is an important part of your life, but regardless of this, if you find that the dog or cat that sleeps in your room or on your bed often wakes you up during the night, then consider whether, for your own sake, you need to get them to sleep in another room. One participant in my sleep clinic online course confessed that three cats slept on her bed, and yes, they did wake her up throughout the night.

If you have a partner who snores, once you've ruled out the possibility that they may suffer from sleep apnea (see page 33), there are various approaches you can adopt. We tend to snore when we are lying on our back, so try asking them to sleep on their side, wedging a pillow behind them to stop them rolling back into the supine position.

You can also get your partner to learn a particular way of singing that has been found to diminish some kinds of snoring by exercising the larynx. See the Resources section for the link. Or you could try getting a Smart Nora, a neat device that uses a microphone by the bed to detect any snoring. When it does, it inflates a balloon under the pillow that tips the snorer's head in another direction. This really does the trick, but it won't work well if you both snore, because the microphone won't know whose snores it's picking up.

You can try various products from the pharmacy for snoring relief, such as nose strips and nostril dilators, throat sprays, and lozenges that stick to the roof of your mouth to waft menthol vapours through your nasal passageways—but you might well find that the most effective product is the cheapest. Packs of mouth tapes can be bought online, and these literally tape your mouth closed. I've tried them, and strangely enough, I found I got used to them quite quickly and my partner reported a marked reduction in my snoring.

The snoring problem is so ubiquitous you could open a shop with all the products and devices that claim to help. They include mandibular splints that hold your lower jaw forward and a machine you use during the day that electrically stimulates your tongue and windpipe, supposedly retraining those parts of the body to help stop you from snoring.

If you've tried all of these and none of them work, then you might need to ask your snoring friend to sleep in another room—if not permanently, then at least for some nights during the week, perhaps for a trial period to see how it goes. A recent survey found that two-thirds of US households include someone who snores and that more than 40 percent of these have the perpetrator sleeping in a separate bedroom.

The problem with this, of course, is that it can undermine the intimacy of the relationship, but there are work-arounds. You can start off in the same bed for cuddles or sex, then move to your separate bedroom before going to sleep. Or you can make dates. To some this would feel too cold and calculating; to others this could be exciting. See more on snoring in Part Two of this book on page 149.

Much of the advice given in this chapter comes under the rubric of sleep hygiene and is a key component in CBT-I; we've just added a spiritual perspective to it. Let's now imagine that you've followed the advice: You've redecorated your bedroom; perhaps you've treated yourself to a new mattress and a great new memory foam pillow; you've got blackout blinds or thick curtains; and you fitted double glazing so that the room is quieter. You've got some NASA-recommended plants in place, and maybe a rock crystal lamp, too. You've got the smell of lavender in the room, if you like it, and you're ready to go: the ashram, the sanctuary, the temple is prepared! Now all you need are some techniques designed to help you make that journey into the Otherworld, the Land of Nod.

Step 5

Choose Your Medicine
Thirteen Ways to Get to Sleep

*Here you discover a whole range of ways of getting to sleep that
you can mix and match to help you drop into sleep, either as
your night begins or if you wake up in the night and need help
getting back to sleep. And you'll find five of these techniques
demonstrated, along with the scripts they use.*

Time for the juicy stuff: techniques to actually get you to sleep. If
you've been tempted to skip to this section that's understandable, but
do go back to the previous steps once you've looked this through.

Remember you need just three things for a good night's sleep: a
safe, comfortable place to sleep, a calm mind, and a relaxed body. The
methods given here will help calm your mind and relax your body,
but it will be hard for them to be effective if you are in an aroused
state. That's why the work of the previous steps is essential, so that
you do not go to bed overstimulated, and as you are heading towards
a trough, not a peak, in your circadian rhythm.

To use a flying analogy, a successful takeoff requires an aircraft
and an airport that are in good condition. This section of the
book is about take-off, about how to lift off into that other state of
consciousness called sleep. But how successful you are in leaving the
ground, and how long your journey lasts, depends to a great extent
on your aircraft and airport; in other words, your set and setting:

your surroundings and how you are feeling in heart, mind, and body. Preparation is everything, as they say, so Steps 1 to 4 are all about prep. Now you're in the cockpit, and we're going to run through 13 ways you can start taxiing down that runway.

The 13 methods we are going to explore include visualization, listening, tensing and releasing of muscles, breathing, movement, and touch. For some people, moving their bodies as they try to get to sleep will seem counterintuitive; for others, lying still and trying to imagine something will seem hard. Even if a technique seems weird or unlikely to work for you, give it a go—you might be pleasantly surprised.

A few words of caution: It can feel overwhelming to read about all these different ways to get to sleep—which one or combination should you try? My advice is to just read through the description of each method and see if one of the methods speaks to you or resonates with you, then try that for a while and see if it works. If it does, then there's no need to explore the others, unless you're curious.

Alternatively, try this prescription: After following the recommendations in Steps 1 to 4 in this book, program a good night's rest by doing the sophrology exercise on pages 65–66 every morning for a week, then let that go once you're sleeping better. During the same one-week period, in the evening, when you go to bed, if you find it hard to drift off, listen to my *Healing Sleep* or one of the other audios recommended in the Resources Section. If you wake up in the night and find it hard to get back to sleep, either switch on the audio again or do the Autogenic Lateral Scan, Silva Method visualization, or breathing technique, which are all explained below.

1. CBT-I: Cognitive Behavioural Therapy for Insomnia aka Behavioural Sleep Medicine

I mentioned in the Introduction that my approach in this book would be to combine the evidence-based, scientifically validated treatments for insomnia with alternative approaches that have not yet been proven to work but that many people find extremely helpful.

Cognitive Behavioural Treatment for Insomnia (CBT-I), sometimes presented as Behavioural Sleep Medicine, alongside the pharmaceutical interventions (sleeping pills and amitryptyline) covered in Step 3, are the only treatments that have gathered enough proof to be considered "evidence-based". Some of the other techniques listed below in this section, such as sophrology and hypnotherapy, have been researched in a limited number of studies, but not enough to gather sufficient proof of their value—at least to the scientific community. Nevertheless, many people report success with these methods.

In clinical research, CBT-I scores slightly higher in effectiveness than sleeping pills, with as many as 70 percent of patients with insomnia experiencing improvements in their condition. This includes waking up less often during sleep, a longer time spent actually sleeping each night, and being able to fall asleep more easily. Both the NHS in the UK and the American College of Physicians in the US recommend that all adult patients complaining of insomnia receive CBT-I as a first-line approach.

What exactly is CBT-I? Cognitive Behavioural Therapy helps people think in more positive ways about their problem and identifies thoughts, feelings, and behaviours that may be causing or exacerbating the issue. With CBT-I, the focus is on looking at ways of "cognitive restructuring" (which simply means changing the way you think) in relation to your sleep. You are given psychoeducation in good "sleep hygiene", which again is a complicated way of saying you learn about how sleep works and what practices you can engage in to get better sleep. You are also taught relaxation techniques.

So far, so good. These components are offered in the Six-Step Program given in this book, with each step involving you learning about sleep (psychoeducation). Step 1 invites major cognitive restructuring through reframing, and in Step 5 you are now learning about a number of techniques that, at heart, involve relaxation. The only unique components in CBT-I are particular interventions developed from the Behavioural Psychology school of thought; of these, the two most commonly used are Stimulus Control and Sleep Restriction.

With **Stimulus Control**, the aim is to maximize the positive sleep-related associations with your bedroom and bedtime and eliminate any associations that are negative or non-sleep related. We cover much of this in Step 4, reclaiming the bedroom as a tranquil place dedicated to drifting off, but in addition to this, CBT-I Stimulus Control asks you to follow these rules: (1) Go to bed only when sleepy; (2) Wake up at the same time every morning; (3) Use the bed only for sleep or sex (that is, no reading, watching TV, and so forth in the bedroom); (4) Avoid excessive napping during the day; and (5) Get out of bed if you are unable to sleep.

If you follow the advice on pages 35–39 about knowing when to go to sleep and wake up in accordance with your circadian rhythm, and how much sleep you need, following rules 1 and 2 should be easy; rule 3 is straightforward, and for rule 4, see page 106 about napping.

It's Rule 5 that's the tricky one. One client described it to me as "brutal", particularly if you live in a cold flat and have to force yourself to get up.

How long can you stay warm in bed? Protocols vary, but here's the instruction to the patient for this rule given in one paper:

> If you find yourself unable to fall asleep, get up and go into another room. Stay up as long as you wish and then return to the bedroom to sleep. Although we do not want you to watch the clock, we want you to get out of bed if you do not fall asleep immediately. Remember, the goal is to associate your bed with falling asleep *quickly!* If you are in bed more than about 10 minutes without falling asleep and have not gotten up, you are not following this instruction. If you still cannot fall asleep, repeat this step as often as is necessary throughout the night.[1]

In the context of this section of the Six-Step Program, which offers 13 ways to help you get off to sleep once you're in bed, you might like to try this technique of getting up for a while if you're not starting to drift off after 10 minutes or so.

If you think this is tough, remember this technique works well for a lot of people, and it's not nearly as tough as the next technique that

CBT-I uses, which ramps up that rule about having to get out of bed if you're not sleeping. It's known as **Sleep Restriction**.

The idea behind Sleep Restriction comes from the observation that people with insomnia often spend a lot of time lying in bed awake: before initially falling asleep, having woken up in the night, then in the morning after waking up. Sleep Restriction involves eliminating virtually all time in bed that is not spent sleeping.

To use this technique, you have to calculate the total time spent asleep on a typical night by using a sleep diary for a week or so. Then the time you allow yourself in bed is controlled to reflect this amount, with a 30-minute bonus to give you some leeway. In other words, if you only sleep for five hours a night and toss and turn while awake for the other three hours you lie in bed, you are asked to restrict your time in bed to five and a half hours. Initially, this procedure tends to increase the fatigue you experience during the day, but that's the point. Gradually, with the help of your CBT-I therapist or online training, you will increase the time you sleep in bed to six hours, and so on, until you get to the time you need—usually seven, eight, or nine hours.

CBT-I is indeed tough and requires discipline, but it really does succeed in curing insomnia for a lot of people by teaching good sleep habits, ways to stop unhelpful thought patterns and reframing how you relate to sleep, and a technique to help you relax—typically, Progressive Muscle Relaxation, which is detailed in this section.

2. Sophrology

Sophrology is huge in the French-speaking world but so far virtually unknown in the English-speaking one. It came to France over 60 years ago, when a Colombian neuro-psychiatrist, Professor Alfonso Caycedo, began researching how he could combine techniques drawn from modern psychology and physiology with the meditative practices of Buddhism and yoga. Fellow doctors joined him in developing the technique, and over the coming years, sophrology evolved to include insights and techniques found in a range of disciplines, including hypnosis, mindfulness, CBT, and NLP.

In France and Switzerland, sophrology is flourishing and being taught to cancer patients, victims of PTSD, expectant mothers, and adults and children suffering from anxiety. It is also popular with sportspeople hoping to emulate the results achieved by Dr. Raymond Abrezol, who coached the Swiss Olympic team using sophrology with startling success and a number of gold medals.

It's essentially a system of brief exercises that take fewer than 15 minutes a day and make use of the nervous system's amazing ability to rewire itself through the process known as neuroplasticity. The exercises use light physical movement, breathing, and visualization to reduce stress and enhance confidence and trust in life. It's particularly good for helping people sleep.

Let me offer you one sophrology exercise that can prove effective; in essence, it programs you for a better night's sleep. You do not do this exercise when preparing for bed; you do it during the day, at any time, and it takes 10–15 minutes. Some people find that simply doing it once is sufficient, but you can do it as often as you like, and it's best to try it daily for a week or so. It involves going into a state of deep relaxation. In this state, you visualize yourself preparing to go to bed, brushing your teeth, and so on, and then, for a while, you imagine yourself having a really good night's sleep. Then you see yourself waking up in the morning, feeling bright and refreshed. That's it.

On first learning about this technique, I was sceptical. It seemed too simplistic. But it's a favourite exercise of the people who take my sleep clinic course—they find it really effective. That's because it works in the same way that certain sports psychology exercises work: By rehearsing success in an activity, you're making it easier for your nervous system and consciousness to replicate the experience, creating new neural pathways. It's also effective because sophrology makes use of an induction technique that gets you into an altered state, thereby making you more suggestible. In order to get you into this deeply relaxed state, it uses a combination of a body scan and what is known as a tension release. You can find the full script for **programming a good night's rest** on page 82, but here let me give you a summary of what the exercise involves.

You stand directly in front of a chair and close your eyes. You then scan your awareness down your body, from the top of your head to the soles of your feet. Then you take in a big breath. You hold that as you tense all the muscles in your body, then you expel the air from your lungs vigorously while letting out a sigh, imagining all the tension falling away from you. You do that three times, then, with eyes still closed, you sit on the chair.

This technique has the effect of relaxing you deeply, most likely taking you from a normal brain wave state of beta to an alpha brain wave state, signalling a more calm and relaxed mood. You then imagine that you're going through the sequence I've described: visualizing yourself having a good night's sleep. You finish the exercise by gently stretching and coming to a sense of wakefulness, feeling fully present here and now. At this point, if you've got the audio edition of this book, you're at a serious advantage, because it will talk you through this exercise.

When Professor Caycedo developed sophrology, he began by researching hypnosis, and although he believed his sophrology was different and superior in effect, the techniques are undeniably related, so let's look now at hypnotherapy's ability to get you to sleep.

3. Hypnotherapy

Like sophrology, not enough rigorously designed double-blind trials have been conducted to conclusively prove that hypnosis can relieve insomnia, but this applies to all of the methods suggested here, apart from CBT-I. Research is difficult, expensive, and time-consuming.

Most hypnotherapists and sophrologists, on finding their method helps their clients, have just got on with applying it, although there are a few notable exceptions, and their studies are mentioned in the endnotes. I also doubt whether the 43,000 people who have said that they like hypnotherapist Michael Sealey's Sleep Hypnosis offering on Youtube care whether the method he's using has been proven to work or not. That recording has been listened to 5.5 million times.

The Sleep Foundation in the US offers its cautious approval of the method, stating that "by encouraging relaxation and creating an opportunity to reorient thoughts and emotions, hypnosis may be a useful tool in enhancing sleep for people with conditions like insomnia."[2]

If you'd like to try hypnosis to see if it helps, experiment with some of the many offerings available online. Combined with all the prep you've done in Steps 1 to 4 and some sophrology programming, as outlined above, and then enacting the final step in this program, you may well find yourself sleeping better. But if you want an individually tailored experience, you can find plenty of hypnotherapists keen to offer their services.

The well-known British hypnotherapist and self-help guru Paul McKenna offers an interesting application of the hypnotic technique for the problem suffered by many people who can't stop their brains running in overdrive when they lie down at night. He points out that most of us "talk to ourselves"—that we have a kind of internal voice speaking our thoughts to ourselves. We might "beat ourselves up" in a critical voice likely to be that of an internalized parent or teacher, or we might "chatter" to ourselves nervously. He has found that when you ask people who are unable to stop thinking or worrying as they lie in bed, they will report an internal voice that tends to speak urgently and negatively: *Why can't I get to sleep? How much longer must I wait?*

McKenna suggests you learn how to **change the tone and pacing of your inner voice**. Remember when you criticized yourself, most likely in a harsh tone of voice? Now imagine giving yourself the same message in a slow, sexy voice. What a difference!

In his book, *I Can Help You Sleep,* McKenna writes that when he examined closely how insomniacs were speaking to themselves:

> I found they were all using some version of an irritated, frustrated, or in some way agitated tone of voice. The pace was also fast. The result was that feelings of irritation or agitation kept them in a physiological state of excitement, which kept them awake.

The solution? When you catch yourself thinking in this way as you lie in bed, practise changing that inner voice and speaking to yourself in a slow, gentle tone of voice. If you listen to hypnotherapists, you'll find they deliver their scripts in a kind of relaxing, tired-sounding, calm, and gentle voice that can seem almost monotonous or boring. Copy them. When you catch yourself worrying or overthinking as you lie in bed, change the tone to sound pleasantly tired and drowsy, "as though the voice can hardly stay awake", as McKenna puts it. You can locate whereabouts you hear it—perhaps in the front of your head, the back of it, or to one side, and then move it a little way away. Then imagine how it might sound quite far away. You can let the voice yawn every few words, ". . . so that [yawn] every few words [yawn], the voice has to stop to yawn [and yawn], and you notice how very delightfully, comfortably tired you feel as you hear those words [yawn] drifting around your awareness."[3]

You could try practising this inner voice by using it to read—to yourself or out loud— the Hypnotherapy for Sleep script you can find on page 85, which was kindly supplied by expert hypnotherapist Mark Tyrell of Uncommon Practitioners and designed to be used if you wake up in the night and find it hard to get back to sleep.

4. The Silva Method

At around the same time Caycedo was developing sophrology in the French-speaking world, an electrical engineer in the US, José Silva, was also studying hypnosis and developing his own method of accessing the altered states of consciousness that sophrology and hypnosis seem to tap into. Soon it became as popular in the US, and in many other countries, as did sophrology in its more limited territory.

The Silva Method is built around a particular technique of self-hypnosis. Once you've used this to get into a relaxed state, you are then able to utilize various techniques for healing, self-development, goal-achievement, and so on. The technique offered for helping you go to sleep is essentially a variation on "counting sheep", designed to **tire your conscious mind** so that it eventually gives up. It can be a helpful way either to tip you into sleep at the beginning of the night or to use if you find yourself awake in the middle of the night.

The technique involves first relaxing yourself. You can use a special Silva method based on auto-hypnosis or another relaxation technique, such as the Autogenic Lateral Scan given in this section.

Once relaxed, imagine yourself in front of a blackboard, with a piece of chalk in one hand and a blackboard eraser in the other hand. Visualize yourself standing in front of the blackboard. Younger readers may be unfamiliar with this teaching aid that was so common in the past, in which case, imagine doing this exercise with a whiteboard and marker pen or with a pencil and paper. We are using the old-fashioned image of a blackboard because the dark background helps evoke a sense of night-time and its associations with sleep.

Have the piece of chalk, pen, or pencil in one hand and the eraser in the other. Imagine approaching the board and drawing a large circle in the centre. Then write a big "X" in the middle of the circle. Now erase the "X", taking great care not to erase any of the circle in the slightest way. To the right of the circle, write the word "DEEPER". (Going forward, whenever you write the word "DEEPER", you enter a *deeper* level of mind, moving *deeper* into sleep.)

Now write the number "100" within the circle. Then slowly erase this number, taking great care not to erase any of the circle in the slightest way. Write over the word "DEEPER", writing the word again on top of the word already written. Every time you write this word, you enter a *deeper* level of mind, moving *deeper* into sleep.

Continue by writing the number "99" within the circle and erasing it in the same manner and then going over the word "DEEPER". Then write "98", "97", and so on, continuing the exercise until you fall asleep.

When you do this exercise, focus on the details: be really careful not to erase the circle in any way; always erase the numbers in the same way, perhaps from left to right or from the centre outwards; go over the word "DEEPER" really slowly and carefully. This focus will help you fall asleep more quickly.

There are endless potential variations on this kind of exercise. One teacher I know who can't bear imagining blackboards imagines the numbers forming out of puffy white clouds against a blue sky. If your mind is racing and you find concentration difficult, it may take you a while to succeed with such an exercise, but you might find that you can gradually develop the focus needed. Or you might prefer just letting go to the sort of guided journey that our next method offers.

5. Yoga Nidra

One of the most effective ways to get to sleep involves using a technique called yoga nidra. Many people will be familiar with the yoga nidra exercise from the end of their hatha yoga session, when the instructor invites them to lie on their yoga mat and takes them through a guided meditation. Often people doze off at this point.

While many people think that yoga nidra is an ancient method, the reality is that it is a combination of ancient yogic wisdom with a range of techniques and ideas drawn from modern Western psychology and medicine.

Yoga nidra as we know it today was developed by Swami Satyananda in the 1960s and 70s, and his book on the subject was published in 1976. Initially inspired by the tantric practice of Nyasa Kriya, in which attention is gradually moved from one point in the body to another, Satyananda also seems to have been influenced by 1930s "relaxationists" Heinrich Schultz and Edmund Jacobsen, who developed the successful systems of Autogenic training and Progressive Muscle Relaxation, respectively. These systems captured the healing potential of learning how to relax deeply, and we find them still in use today, with autogenic training being used in particular by nurses in hospitals, and progressive relaxation being used in CBT-I.

Into the mix, Satyananda added the psychology of Carl Jung and his ideas about archetypal images and symbols, and Emile Coué's ideas on auto-suggestion, and combined all these inspirations into a technique that involves lying down in what is known as Savasana, the yogic Corpse Pose, to begin taking a pilgrimage of consciousness through the body.

Yoga nidra's effectiveness comes from the way it includes a certain kind of body scan which, rather than being the sweep of awareness with which you may be familiar from mindfulness meditation, invites you instead to move your attention around your body on a particular route. This has the effect of being very soporific.

In addition to that, it invites you to breathe in certain ways and work with imagery and experiences of opposite sensations or concepts, such as light and dark, hot and cold, high and low. This also has an extremely soporific effect, helping your consciousness change gear and loosening the grip of your rational mind. If the act of lying down and following directions to move your awareness in a route that eventually covers almost every part of your body hasn't already sent you to sleep, these techniques of consciously breathing in special ways and becoming aware of opposite qualities will generally do the trick.

In recent years, a number of people have developed their own varieties of yoga nidra, including the American psychologist Dr. Richard Miller, whose iRest system is now used in many clinical settings. There are many yoga nidras available online (see the Resources section for recommendations, and choose the recording with the voice, pacing, and style that suits you best). To give you a sense of what you are invited to do as you listen to a yoga nidra, see the sample script given on page 88. This may send you to sleep just reading it— it's not exactly boring, but you'll see what I mean!

The great advantage of using yoga nidras as your means of getting to sleep is that if you don't go to sleep, you will have the most wonderful adventures in consciousness; it's a win/win situation. If you're someone who wakes up after a few hours of sleep and then takes hours and hours to get back to sleep, if you do a long yoga nidra, you will be having a very deep meditative experience, whether you sense yourself as asleep or not. In this way, you will be truly accepting the gift of the night, really working with this idea of the night being a time of spiritual retreat—a time when you can not only restore yourself with deep relaxation but also be inspired by some of the very deepest sources of spiritual inspiration.

6. Tapping: the Emotional Freedom Technique (EFT)

There's something about moving your awareness from place to place around the body that can induce a sleepy state, and this next method makes use of the same mechanism we've seen at work in yoga nidra with the additional feature of using physical movement as well as the imagination.

Tapping, or the Emotional Freedom Technique (EFT), was developed in the 1970s. It involves tapping one's fingers at acupuncture points along body "meridians", the purported channels that carry life force through the body, while simultaneously thinking about an issue or repeating affirmations. You can find short videos online taking you through EFT tapping routines for insomnia, which usually involve starting by tapping the side of the hand repeatedly for about 40 seconds before moving to the top of the head, tapping gently a few times, then moving down via various points on the face and chest, and finishing by placing both hands flat against the chest. Variations of this sequence exist, but all seem to cover this upper area of the body.

As you tap, some practitioners recommend you repeat affirmations such as "I choose to get a good night's sleep", "I choose to love and accept myself", "I choose to fall asleep easily", "I choose to fall asleep quickly", and so on. Apparently, using the paradoxical intention technique, mentioned on page 26, can work well, too: With this you say the reverse of a positive affirmation: "I can't get to sleep." With this variation, some people promptly fall asleep, or so practitioners recount. Perhaps this works through "reverse psychology", engaging some people's feelings of defiance, or perhaps it simply demonstrates the relaxing power of acceptance and letting go of trying to force change.

EFT proponents also suggest that you can simply imagine yourself tapping at the various points as you recount the affirmations. Lying in bed with eyes closed, you go through the routine in your mind, essentially performing a variation of the "pilgrimage around the body" of yoga nidra but imagining tapping at the stopping points, too, and adding the use of affirmations.

7. Progressive Muscle Relaxation

Relax your right arm. Notice how this feels. Now tense up all the muscles in that arm as you hold your breath. Now let go of that tension as you breathe out. It's likely that now your arm feels even more relaxed. This is the basis of the Progressive Muscle Relaxation technique: you do this throughout the body, progressing up or down it, hence the term "progressive".

Of all the techniques given in this section of the book, this is the favourite of my very active grandson Leo, who at the age of 10, like many modern kids the same age, usually goes to sleep with the aid of his smartphone or iPad. It's a favourite of CBT-I therapists, too, although quite a range of different techniques can be used in CBT-I, according to the preference of the practitioner.

They all come under the umbrella term of Relaxation Training, and in addition to progressive muscle relaxation, which was developed in the 1930s, they include autogenic training, biofeedback, self-hypnosis, and meditation techniques. I predict that eventually many CBT-I therapists will include sophrology and yoga nidra in their repertoires. You can find a script for this method on page 91.

8. The Autogenic Lateral Scan

You may well be familiar with the concept of a body scan from mindfulness or other kinds of meditation. Just running your awareness slowly down or up your body can be very relaxing and is often a useful preparation at the start of a meditation session. Yoga nidras use a variation on this technique by asking you instead to move your attention from point to point, or area to area, around your body.

It's often hard to stay awake on these pilgrimages around the body as you lie on a yoga mat or bed, nicely snug with pillows and a blanket. If you do them a lot, you can eventually lead yourself without a recording, having learnt the "pilgrimage routes". This is a handy strategy if you wake up at night and don't want to move to switch on a recording, but most people find that allowing someone else to lead the journey makes it easier for the conscious mind to "switch off" and fall asleep.

But here's a variation on this idea, partly inspired by a system called Autogenic training. Developed in the 1920s, it was favoured by health professionals, particularly nurses, though it's gone a little out of fashion now.

It's essentially a variation on the normal body scan, with the addition of a rather effective technique of becoming aware of the weight, size, and temperature of each limb. And instead of sweeping up or down your body the way it is usually done with a body scan, it involves scanning one leg, then flipping over in your awareness to scan the other leg, then flipping across to scan one arm, and then across to scan the other arm, and then down the torso. Each time before you flip, you spend a few moments getting a sense of the temperature, weight, and size of the area you've just scanned. This may sound like a lot of work, but it isn't! A lot of people find it's the only technique they need to drop off. You'll find the full instructions for this exercise later on in this section.

9. The Power of Sound to Help You Sleep

We are so lucky these days. With access to the internet, we can find out whether certain kinds of music or spoken word, white noise, binaural beats, or ASMR recordings can help us nod off. We can set up our smartphone or tablet to play for hours and create our own playlists. So if you find that listening to the radio, podcasts, or music often helps, it's worth looking at this way of getting to sleep in more detail.

The problem with listening to audiobooks, a radio station, or a podcast is that you can never quite be sure that you won't be woken by a sudden noise or change of tone, a chilling announcement about some awful breaking news, or simply something unusual or fascinating that catches your attention as you cycle from deep sleep into light sleep, when you reach that peak of alertness in your circadian rhythm mentioned on page 36.

If this happens for you, try creating a playlist of music that you know is soothing and has no sudden switches in tone or occasional clash of cymbals or blast of trumpets. You could try the composer Max Richter's eight-hour-long composition, which has been played to live audiences tucked up in sleeping bags all over the world.

When I had insomnia, I decided to capitalize on the idea of the "gift of the night" offering a mini spiritual retreat, and I created a playlist of Western and Eastern sacred music—John Taverner, Gorecki, Arvo Pärt—with chants from the great traditions of India, too. If I woke up at any time, I could just enjoy their numinous beauty. Nowadays, you can find great playlists on Spotify. Have a look at the ones for psychedelic therapy sessions. Because these sessions tend to go on for hours, the playlists are long and often very soothing.

If you prefer the human voice to music, there are podcasts of "bedtime stories for adults" that are deliberately designed to avoid being overly interesting, and nothing frightening or even exciting happens in the stories. A particular favourite for people who take our sleep clinic is *NothingMuchHappens.com* or you could try the Sleep Stories section in the Calm app.

Other people prefer natural sounds to the human voice or music: the sound of rain outside, the sea or wind, or even a storm. Apps such as Infinite Storm will provide you with many variations on this theme.

A favourite device I use for afternoon naps (but which can also be used for sending you to sleep at night) is a sophrology machine called the Morphée, which sits by your bed and plays a variety of music, sounds, and spoken sophrology relaxation routines.

Some people find that the consistent ambient masking effect of white noise (which you could compare to the sound of a fan or air conditioner humming away) helps them sleep, but in fact, you can now access a whole range of "sonic hues", and it's just a question of finding the one that suits you best. Go online and you can find eight-hour long recordings of White, Pink, Blue, Violet, Red, Brown, Grey, Green, Orange, and Black Noise. White noise makes use of all the frequencies available to the human ear, whereas the different coloured variations alter this mix. Pink noise has reduced higher frequencies, brown noise even fewer, and so on.

Or perhaps what are known as "binaural beats" will help. These beats are a perception of sound created by your brain when tones of different frequencies are played in each ear. If you listen to a tone at 300 hertz (Hz) in one ear, for example, and to a tone at 310 Hz in the other, the binaural beat you will hear is at 10 Hz. Early research is suggesting that listening to recordings that generate binaural beats may help reduce anxiety and lead to improved sleep, with one study finding that the restorative phase of deep sleep was lengthened in participants exposed to them. Again, you can find many recordings online, including recordings that combine binaural beats with the white or coloured noises mentioned above.

You might also like to find out whether you are susceptible to ASMR (autonomous sensory meridian response). If you are, you will find that certain sounds or images make you feel very relaxed and generate pleasurable tingling feelings in your head and neck. Research hasn't determined how many of us have this ASMR response, but judging by the YouTube viewing figures it must be a good proportion. If you're not susceptible, the videos seem strange, even a bit spooky. Someone will be simply folding towels or pretending to brush your hair. Running water and even sounds like rustling plastic or scratching nails along a hard surface can generate the experience for some people.

ASMR can be seen as the opposite experience to misophonia, which afflicts those who are extremely sensitive to certain sounds, such as chewing or breathing, and trigger intense feelings of anger, agitation, and disgust. Interestingly, a large-scale study of misophonia found that half the participants also experienced ASMR, and other research has found differences in neural connectivity and networking amongst those reporting ASMR.[4,5]

Most people with ASMR use the experience to help them get to sleep, and you can find a vast range of videos online, including role-playing "sleep doctor exams", which have millions of viewings, with at least one video lasting three hours. How do they help people sleep? No one yet knows for certain, but those with ASMR find that the experience lifts their mood, relieves anxiety, and induces relaxation and calm: all important ingredients for easing our entry into the world of dreams. The National Sleep Foundation in the US recommends ASMR University as a good resource.

10. Breathing

Google (or better still, use the eco-friendly search engine Ecosia) for methods for getting to sleep fast, and you'll soon find the popular health guru Andrew Weil, a Harvard doctor, sharing with you the **4–7–8 breathing technique** that he has taken from yoga and popularized. It involves breathing in for four counts, holding for seven and breathing out for eight. By doing this, you're altering the oxygenation levels in your body in a way that is soothing and calming to your physiology. It's very simple to do, and for some people it works like a dream, sending them straight off to sleep.

If you find it doesn't work on its own, try combining it with another technique. A good combination is to try it with the autogenic scan, using the breathing technique before you begin the scan. Or try the following either during or after the 4-7-8 breathing exercise: As you breathe in, move your eyes so that behind the lids they are looking upwards. As you breathe out, feel yourself relaxing as you move your eyes to look downwards. Breathe in . . . and your eyes float up; breathe out . . . and your eyes move gently down as you let go. Feel yourself dropping down into the bed, relaxing even more deeply.

11. Jin Shin Jyutsu

Studies have found that acupuncture and acupressure can help people sleep better. The central idea behind these therapies is that life force flows in channels called meridians and that if this flow can be freed of blockages and harmonized, good health and improved sleep will follow.

A number of modalities offer techniques based on this idea to help you drift into sleep, including EFT, Havening, and Jin Shin Jyutsu.

Jin Shin Jyutsu was developed in Japan at around the same time that shiatsu was created, in the early 20th century. Jin Shin Jyutsu, which means literally "the Creator's art through the compassionate person", uses a simpler model of meridians than acupuncture and shiatsu, and is also inspired by the use of different hand positions to achieve different states of consciousness, known as *mudras* in Buddhist practice.

Jin Shin Jyutsu offers a healing system you can self-administer or use on others. It is relatively simple and involves placing your hands on particular areas of your body for 3–5 minutes, although you can continue the hold for up to 20 minutes if you wish. Just placing your fingertips, fingers, or palms at these points while you assume a relaxed attitude of receiving is said to be sufficient.

The gentle healing art of using the hands for healing and self-healing in this way is perhaps best demonstrated by taking one of your hands and placing your palm against your sternum, at the centre of your chest, or try it on a friend. How does it feel? Most likely, soothing and comforting.

Jin Shin Healing Touch: Quick Help for Common Ailments by Tina Stümpfig provides clear instructions on how to use this technique, which for insomnia involves touching three points.

1 As you lie in bed, ready to fall asleep, place one hand over the inside of the other hand and hold the fleshy pad at the base of the thumb for 3–20 minutes. Then do the same thing on the other hand.

2 Next, turning the hand on its side with the thumb in the air, grasp the thumb with your fingers and hold it, again for 3 minutes or more. Do the same on the other hand.

3 Finally, if you are still awake, keeping your hand in the sideways position with the thumb in the air, place the other hand behind it for support and lay your thumb across the base of the fingers above the palm, and hold this position, again for 3 minutes or more. Then do the same on the other hand.

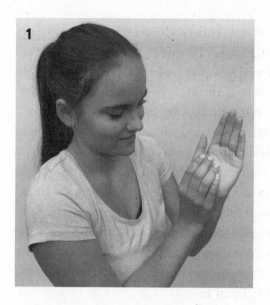

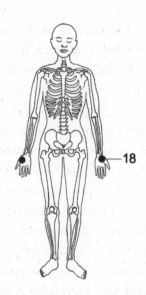

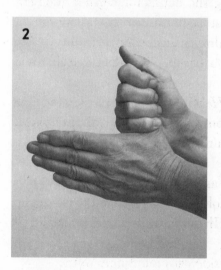

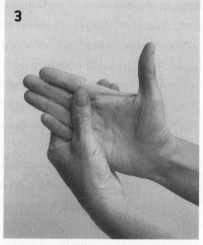

Adopting an open-minded attitude of relaxed curiosity is probably the best approach to trying out this technique. Jin Shin Jyutsu practitioners encourage you to persevere with the method for some time, since it may be a while before you see the results. A number of instructional videos are viewable online that demonstrate its use for insomnia.

12. Havening

The touch of a hand can be reassuring and soothing. The Jin Shin Jyutsu method uses the power of such touch with a series of mudra-like hand holds. The EFT method uses the fingers of the hand in a very different way to tap the upper body at certain points, finishing with a soothing gesture of resting the hands on the chest. In the Havening method the hands are also used, and like EFT, just on the upper body: the face, head, and upper arms.

Steven and Donald Ruden, the doctor and dentist brothers who developed the havening technique, believe that the use of therapeutic touch can help create a sense of calm and safety within you—a "haven"—and that in this state you can be freed of emotional distress and the symptoms of anxiety and trauma. The Rudens believe that their technique can calm the amygdala, the structure in the brain that is part of the limbic system regulating emotional responses, and also that it can generate the delta brain waves that occur during deep sleep.

Trained practitioners can be found online, but havening is something you can practise on your own. The technique combines gentle stroking with distraction techniques, such as visualization, eye movement, or even singing. A practitioner will ask you to rate your current level of distress on a scale of 1 to 10, then might invite you to stroke your arms and face as you visualize a beautiful scene, or move your eyes from left to right or in a circle. Then they might ask you to hum a tune as they stroke your forehead or arms, or if you'd prefer them not to touch you, you can do this yourself. Finally, you rate your current emotional state, which may well have now improved. Only a few studies have been carried out on this method, but they seem promising.

To practise **self-havening** as a technique for getting to sleep, try this: As you lie in bed, cross your arms as if giving yourself a hug, and slowly and gently stroke your upper arms with your hands as you tell yourself *I am tired, I am drowsy.* Keep doing this, soaking in the feelings of self-care and love, for 5–10 minutes, or until you want to stop and begin to drift off. Look online for videos on this technique, including Dr. Kate Truitt's variation on self-havening, which adds in breathing exercises.

13. The Day Review

I'll finish this section with a method that works for me every time. It's based on a concept found in Rudolf Steiner's spiritual teachings that recommends reviewing your day each evening to help you progress in self-awareness. In addition to any spiritual benefit this exercise might provide, from a psychological perspective it makes sense that undigested experience may become unsettling and provoke anxiety that inhibits sleep, and that regular reviews of your experience could help process and resolve any challenging feelings and clear your heart and mind, allowing you to drop into sleep more easily.

The technique suggests that, as you lie in bed, settling in for the night, you start replaying the experiences of your day in reverse order. In other words, you start off by thinking about what you did just before you went to bed: brushing your teeth and so on, and then perhaps the TV program you watched and how you enjoyed it and what you learned from it. Then back to the evening meal, thinking about that, and then gradually working back through your day. The extra effort required to reverse the order seems to help in making you sleepy. I very rarely get to revisit what happened that morning, but if I do and I'm still awake, I just keep going, by trying to recall the previous day's experiences.

This technique works well with most forms of gratitude practice. Psychologists have found that calling to mind the positive experiences of our day and focusing on feelings of gratitude is beneficial, and you can easily add this practice in to your day review.

The Day Review technique is probably not advised if you've had a traumatic or really upsetting day, and some people, particularly if they have a tendency to sleep procrastination (see page 119), report that revisiting their day makes them worry and awakens their judgmental self, which begins to criticise them for what they did or did not do. If you find that's the case, this technique isn't for you!

Any one of these 13 methods might be just right for you, and you may never need to try any of the others. But psychologists have borrowed a nice musical term for a group of ways to effect change:

they talk about learning a "repertoire of techniques", and if you've made it through this chapter this is what you've just done. Reframing any sleep difficulty you have, not as a problem but as a challenge that requires an adventurous, curious, and solutions-oriented approach, means that even if you've found one of these techniques works like a treat, you might like to try the others, too, if only out of a sense of scientific curiosity. And also, given that a third of adults report sleep difficulties, you might well find yourself able to help a friend by telling them about these methods.

Five Scripts to Practice With

In this section, you'll find scripts for five of the methods I've mentioned. Reading them will give you a sense of how each one works. You could make your own recordings of these, or if you have the audiobook version, you can try them out straight away.

The first exercise is not designed to send you to sleep and is carried out when you are wide awake. If you want to use the other exercises to get to sleep, remember "Set and Setting", as laid out in detail in Steps 1 to 4 of this program.

If you are feeling wired, wide awake, anxious, or troubled, these methods may start the process of helping you let go and unwind, but they might not send you to sleep. For these scripts to really work, make sure that you have carried out the preparatory work, and that you are in, or moving towards, a trough in your circadian rhythm as described on page 36.

✳ Sophrology: Programming a Good Night's Rest ✳

Do this exercise during the day. It's not supposed to send you to sleep; it's designed to reprogram your nervous system so that it guides you automatically into having a good night's rest. Try this exercise several times at least, to give it time to work on your unconscious and on your body. Ideally, do it every day for a week or more—it takes less than 15 minutes.

1   Make sure you have a chair directly behind you. This needs
    to be the sort of chair you would find in the kitchen, dining
    room, or office, not an armchair, which will be too low. Start
    by standing upright, legs about shoulders' distance apart, knees
    relaxed, eyes closed to better concentrate on yourself. Now
    take your awareness outside the room, and see if you can hear
    any sounds from far away. Now move your awareness to any
    sounds inside the room. Now to any sounds that you might be
    hearing from within your own body, such as your digestion, your
    heartbeat, or your breathing.

2   After a few moments, take a deep breath in through the nose
    and down into the abdomen. Hold it for a while and then
    breathe out. Do this twice more.

3   And now move your attention down your body, as if you are
    scanning it, just slowly sweeping your awareness from the top
    of your head to the soles of your feet. Make this as effortless
    as possible. You don't have to try to relax your muscles as you
    do this, although this may well happen. Just allow into your
    awareness whatever you are sensing and feeling, and when you
    have got to the soles of your feet, shift your focus of attention
    to being aware of your whole body.

4   Keep your eyes closed, and breathe in deeply as you sweep
    your arms up, joining your hands together above your head.
    Hold your breath in, and try to tense as many muscles in your
    body as you can. When you can't keep the breath in any longer,
    let it all out with a big sigh as you simultaneously lower your
    arms. Release, relax, let go! Do this twice more. Keeping your
    eyes closed, feel for the chair behind you, and gently lower
    yourself onto it, so you are sitting comfortably with your back
    upright. Take a few moments to let your body settle. Try not
    to think of anything; instead, just be open to any sensations you
    are experiencing.

5   Now imagine that it is the evening. See yourself getting ready
    for bed, brushing your teeth, and so on, doing whatever you
    do for your bedtime routine. Follow the sequence through:

See yourself getting undressed and then climbing into bed and turning out the light.

6   Now fully identify with yourself lying there in the bed—You feel your head and your body in a really comfortable position. You feel the softness and the firmness of the mattress beneath you, the pillow beneath your head . . . Just sense your mind and body relaxing completely . . . starting to let go.

7   Choose a word that is soothing and soporific for you, such as "sleep" or "drift" or "calm", and start to say it to yourself every time you exhale. So sense yourself now, breathing in and breathing out, and every time you breathe out you say the word. Every time you say the word you can sense yourself drifting off to sleep . . . Now see yourself lying in bed. You're looking down on yourself in bed, and you see how comfortable you look. You see how you are sleeping deeply . . . you see yourself going through the different cycles of sleep . . . sometimes shifting in the bed, but sleeping deeply . . . and you watch and sense your body being warm and comfortable . . . your cells relaxed and regenerating . . . your mind relaxed and open to dreaming . . . and you have an inner knowing that all is well . . . you feel this confidence and this feeling of security doing something that occurs naturally every night . . . an essential process that is strengthening and reinforcing your body and mind.

8   And now you see yourself slowly waking up at just the right time . . . You've had such a good night's sleep you're waking up feeling really refreshed . . . and you find yourself looking forward to the day . . . You experience yourself stretching, getting out of bed feeling well and rested . . . and you are looking forward to the day . . . You sense yourself going through the day full of energy, thanks to the peaceful and regenerating night's sleep you've just had. And you know that by regularly doing this exercise your sleep will become more peaceful, more regenerative, your body and your brain will function more efficiently, and you will be more alert and

able to make better decisions . . . and you now let go of the visualization, becoming aware of your body seated on the chair, feeling completely relaxed.

9   Let your awareness settle for a few moments, just aware of any sensations you might be experiencing in your body. Then finish the exercise with the following affirmation, as you consciously breathe in and out, deeply and slowly:

With each breath, I feel a deep sense of confidence and trust in myself; I feel my mind and body, my heart and soul, completely harmonized. With each breath I am creating a positive future for myself, filled with happiness and wellbeing.

Stretch your fingers and toes, and when you feel ready, in your own time, open your eyes. When in bed at night, you can take the word you chose at Step 7 to help you drift off, mentally saying it for as long as you want, every time you breathe out.

✳ Hypnotherapy for Sleep ✳

This script, created by master hypnotherapist Mark Tyrell of Uncommon Practitioners, needs to be spoken slowly in a relaxing, tired-sounding, calm voice that can seem almost monotonous, with plenty of pauses.

Now the deep relaxation technique you're about to experience mimics the process your brain naturally follows to drift off to sleep comfortably and easily, each and every night, because it increasingly shifts your attention from focusing on the external world to being able to focus fully inside on the images and landscapes of your imagination, as you begin to relax deeply and dream. And when you drift off to sleep, it's not as if you switch off your mind; it's that you activate different parts of your brain while your conscious mind can just float into a dream. Your unconscious can heal the body and process the learnings of the day, and here and now, you can pick a spot in the room that you can comfortably gaze at, and if you've closed your eyes you can just gently let them open for a few moments, and even if it's dark you can just gaze at a particular place on the wall or ceiling . . . that's it . . . and really get a sense of that spot, just there . . . that's it . . . And then you can just close those eyes, and imagine what it would be like to mentally zoom in on that spot to magnify it in your mind, and even get a feel for the texture of it. And then you can just let your eyes open once again, and just gaze towards that spot once more, and as you continue to gaze steadily at that spot, you can notice three things you can see in your field of vision. So as your eyes focus deeply on that spot, you might be aware of an object in the room, perhaps a piece of furniture or a patch of light or just a shadow on the wall . . . that's it . . . And when you've noticed three things you can just let those eyes rest closed.

And really beginning to relax deeply now, with those eyes comfortably closed, as you begin to listen to three things you can hear, and now pay attention to three particular sounds . . . like any noises from outside, perhaps the wind or the sound of your breathing or the ticking of a clock . . . just noticing that right now, as you relax deeper still. And then just paying attention to three things you can feel, whether it's the warmth of the bed or the temperature of the air against that face or the sensation of what-ever's supporting that body . . . that's it . . . And you can just keep those eyes firmly and comfortably closed, as you allow that body to relax properly and let that conscious mind begin to drift, as you just imagine what it would be like to open them and look at that spot before you again, but this time you can adjust the time of day it is, even the season it is, and notice how that changes the light, the shadows, the shades of colour . . . that's it . . .

And as you imagine gazing at that spot at a different time and in a different season, you can just notice three new things in your field of vision you can see: another object, a different shadow . . . that's it . . . And then you can just imagine three different sounds you might hear in this different time, different sounds from outside, different weather, or how the sounds might be different in the place where you are now . . . that's it . . . just noticing those three sounds as you continue to drift into deeper comfort. And then you could just notice three things you would feel in this time, a different temperature to the air on that face, the position of that body, the degree of warmth beneath the covers . . . that's it . . .

And as you really relax deeply and fully now and prepare to drift all the way down into deepest sleep, you can just get the sense of what it feels like just before you float into a dream at night, when you get flashes of the images to come, and here and now you could momentarily catch sight of a beautiful green field filled with lush grass rippling in the breeze, just seeing that now for a second and then allowing it to fade, and seeing in its place an ocean sunset and the way the reds, the blues, the oranges, and the pinks all blend together and reflect on the water . . . that's it . . . And then allowing that to fade, and seeing in its place a bird soaring way up into the sky, and just following its movements and the arcs it makes . . . that's it . . .

And there's no need to try, or to try not to try, as your unconscious mind begins to naturally lead you into a deep and comfortable sleep, where you can rest, fully restore, and revitalize. Your energy levels are already charging up, as you drift deeper down and allow that body to do its job, because that body knows how to sleep very well, so here and now you can just pay attention to what waves sound like, as they break on the shore, rhythmically lapping at the sand, lulling you deeper still; what distant, delicate piano music sounds like, gently floating, carried by the wind; what trees sound like, as the wind rustles through their leaves; and you know, do you not, the sensation of touching a tree, and even with your eyes closed, if you gently rubbed the bark of a tree there would be certain rough sensations you would feel, along with a sense of solidity and strength, and if you pulled on one of the thinner branches of a tree you would feel it flex and bend and resist the pull of your hand, and you could even get the sense of rubbing a leaf between those fingertips and feel its cool smoothness . . . that's it . . .

And there are certain animals that know—as winter approaches, as the nights get longer and the days get shorter, and you start to see your breath in the air—that it's time to curl up in their homes and drift into deepest, deepest sleep, and even though there are things happening in the forest and things they could think about, they automatically curl up somewhere snug and safe and fall into a deep state of hibernation, where they sleep ever so deeply. And sometimes, those animals will sleep through storms outside, howling gales and thrashing rain; and sometimes, they will sleep deeply and fully through the storm; other times, they might half-awaken for a moment, only to drift all the way back down into deepest rest, so that when spring comes they have forgotten they ever awoke. And your unconscious can really assist you in being able to sleep deeply and peacefully each and every night . . . that's it . . .

And the more you listen to this, the easier and more natural you will find this, because sleep is an instinctive part of you, so you can just allow it to happen smoothly and naturally. And if you awaken a little, you can forget about it consciously and trust your unconscious is the part of you that knows how you do this instinctively and enter the deepest stages of sleep naturally. And that's it, just floating on the waves of your inner mind and drifting into a dream of what it is, you do not know, yet you can float deeper and deeper still . . .

✳ Yoga Nidra: Body Awareness ✳

Welcome to this practice of yoga nidra. Begin by making yourself comfortable, and as you settle into just the right position for you, be aware that in this session you have no goal. There's no striving. There's nothing you're reaching for. The goal is simply to experience this practice, to enjoy it. The goal isn't to go to sleep or to stay awake. It's possible that you may remain awake, but if you do, the benefits of the exercise will still be present. And you're likely to find it restorative and deeply restful. And if you do find yourself drifting into sleep, you're likely to find your sleep will be deep and restorative, too. And so with no goal in mind, except to enjoy this experience, just get more and more comfortable in the bed, and find a position in which you feel you can remain still. But if you do find yourself wanting to move at any time, just see if you can observe that feeling without acting on it, and it's possible that the feeling will go. But if it doesn't, it's fine to move. Just move if you need to, and then settle back into the experience.

And so now lying here, move your awareness to begin with to any sounds you might hear from outside the room. And if you can hear sounds outside the room, just allow them to be there, just accepting that they're there. And then just moving your attention to any sounds you might hear inside your room. And again, if there are sounds, just accept them. Now move your awareness to sounds you might be experiencing from within your own body. Again, accept any sounds you might hear, and focus now on the sound of your breathing, if you can hear it; and whether you can hear it or not, just focus on your breathing without trying to change it, just becoming aware of it, and just noticing how it occurs effortlessly—the breath flowing into your body and flowing out of your body.

And now move your awareness to the points of contact between your body and the bed. Let's start with the feet: Just move your awareness down to the feet and just sense the feeling of your feet, of being in contact with the mattress, with the bed. And then that sense of contact with the legs and thighs on the mattress, the hips and the back, the shoulder blades, the neck, and the head. You can sense your body resting on the bed and just open to an awareness of its weight—a sense of the weight of the body, its heaviness. Just allow your body to nestle into the bed, as if it's drifting down, sinking down, feeling heavy, sensing the effect of gravity on the body, and just being aware of this sense of gravity, of heaviness. It's possible you might somewhere inside that feeling have a sense of lightness, too, of drifting like a feather.

And now we're going to take a journey of awareness around the body. All you have to do is become aware of the part of the body, as it's mentioned, no need to even try to relax as each part is mentioned, though that may happen. Just move your awareness there. You might want to say the word, or you might want to visualize the part of the body, or you may simply be there in your awareness.

So start by moving your awareness to the right thumb, index finger, middle finger, ring finger, little finger. Then become aware of all the fingers and the thumb together. Now move your awareness to the back of the hand, the palm of the hand, the wrist, the forearm, the elbow, the upper arm, the shoulder, the armpit, the right ribs, the right waist, the right hip, the thigh, the knee, the shin and calf, the ankle, the heel, the top of the foot, the sole of the foot, the right big toe, second toe, third toe, fourth toe, fifth toe, all toes of the right foot.

Now move your awareness to the left thumb, index finger, middle finger, ring finger, little finger, all the fingers and thumb of the left hand. The back of the hand, the palm, wrist, forearm, elbow, the upper arm, the shoulder, the armpit, the left ribs, the left waist, the left hip, thigh, knee, shin, calf, ankle, heel, top of the foot, sole of the foot, left big toe, second toe, third toe, fourth toe, fifth toe.

Become aware of the whole of the left side of the body; now the whole of the right side of the body. Become aware of your right leg, and now become aware of your left leg; both legs together. Become aware of your right arm, become aware of your left arm; both arms together. Move your awareness to your lower back, middle back, upper back, your left shoulder, your right shoulder, the back of the neck, the back of the head, the top of the head, your forehead, the left temple, the right temple, the left eyebrow, the right eyebrow, the left eyelid, the right eyelid. The left eye, the right eye, the left cheek, the right cheek, the bridge of the nose, the tip of the nose, the upper lip, the lower lip, the place where the lips meet, the chin, the neck, the chest, the navel, the front of the body, the back of the body, the whole body, the whole body, the whole body.

And in becoming aware of the whole body, you sense how heavy your body feels. You sense the weight of the body. You sense the heaviness of the body. And now you let go of that, of the sense of heaviness, and you open instead to a sense of lightness—as if it's as light as a feather, floating on the breeze. And feeling that sense of lightness, see if you can also open at the same time to the sense of heaviness. Just invite the possibility that these opposite feelings can coexist within your experience: heavy and light.

And you move your awareness to the breath, just allowing it to flow in and to flow out. And as it flows out, you imagine the breath just flowing down the spine. And as you breathe in, you sense it flowing up the spine. As you breathe out, down the spine, as you breathe in, up the spine. And you do this for as long as you wish, just resting quietly, breathing in and breathing out, allowing your body to rest, feeling deep peace—just being here for as long as you wish.

✳ Progressive Muscle Relaxation ✳

Begin by finding a comfortable position to sit or lie down in. Make sure that you are comfortable. Let your hands rest loosely in your lap or by your side. And, if you are comfortable, gently close your eyes. Become aware of your breathing, and notice how your abdomen rises and falls with each breath . . . Now take a long, slow, deep breath in through your nose, all the way down into your stomach. Hold the breath for just a moment and then exhale through your mouth. Allow your breath to carry away all stress and tension as the air flows out of your lungs. Take another slow breath in through your nose. Fill your lungs completely. Hold it for a moment . . . and release the breath through your mouth. Empty your lungs completely with your out-breath. Take a third deep breath in. Hold it for a moment, and then let it go. Feel that your body has already undergone a change. The tension in your body has begun to loosen and subside. Now let your breathing rhythm return to normal . . . and relax . . . During this relaxation, I will ask you to tense various muscles throughout your body. Please do this without straining; no need to exert yourself, just contract each muscle firmly but gently as you breathe in. If you feel uncomfortable at any time, simply relax and breathe normally.

Bring your awareness to your feet and toes. Breathe in deeply through your nose, and as you do, gradually curl your toes down and tense the muscles in the soles of your feet. Hold your breath for just a few seconds . . . and then release the muscles in your feet as you breathe out. Feel the tension in your feet wash away as you exhale. Notice how different your feet feel when tensed and when they are relaxed.

Take another deep breath in again, tense the muscles in the soles of your feet, and hold this position for a few seconds. Now release. Feel yourself relaxing more and more deeply with each breath. Your whole body is becoming heavier, softer, and more relaxed as each moment passes. Now bring your awareness to your lower legs, to your calf muscles. As you draw in a nice deep breath, point your toes up towards your knees, and tighten these muscles. Hold for just a moment . . . and then let those muscles go limp as you exhale.

Once again, draw in a deep breath . . . and tighten your calf muscles. Hold for a few seconds . . . and then let it all go. Feel your muscles relax, and feel the tension washing away with your out-breath.

Now take a deep breath in, and tense the muscles in your thighs. Hold for just a moment . . . and then release everything. As you do this, the blood flow to your muscles increases and you may notice a warm, tingling sensation. Enjoy this feeling of soothing relaxation in your thighs. Again, breathe in deeply, and tighten your thigh muscles. Hold for a moment . . . now release. Focus on letting your muscles go limp and loose. Draw in a nice deep breath, and gradually tighten the muscles in your buttocks. Hold this contraction for a few seconds . . . and then release your breath. Feel the tension leaving your muscles. Feel them relaxing completely. Once more, breathe in deeply, and tighten the muscles in your buttocks. Hold for a moment . . . now release them. You are becoming more and more deeply relaxed. Take another breath, and this time, gradually tighten all the muscles in your legs, from your feet to your buttocks. Do this in whatever way feels natural and comfortable to you. Hold it . . . and now release all these large, strong muscles. Enjoy the sensation of release as you become even more deeply relaxed.

Now bring your awareness to your stomach. Draw in a nice deep breath and then tighten these muscles. Imagine you are trying to touch your belly button to your spine. Now release your breath, and let your muscles relax. Notice the sensation of relief that comes from letting go. Once again, draw in a deep breath and then tighten your stomach muscles. Hold for a few seconds . . . and then let them relax as you exhale and release all tension.

Bring your awareness to the muscles in your back. As you slowly breathe in, arch your back slightly and tighten these muscles . . . Now release your breath, and let your muscles relax. Again, draw in a deep breath and then tighten your back muscles. Hold for a few seconds . . . and then let them relax and release. Now give your attention to your shoulder muscles and the muscles in your neck. As you slowly draw in a nice deep breath, pull your shoulders up towards your ears, and squeeze these muscles firmly. Now breathe out completely, and allow your contracted muscles to go loose and limp. Again, pull your shoulders up towards your ears, and squeeze these muscles firmly. Now feel the tension subside as you relax and breathe out. Feel the heaviness in your body now. Enjoy the feeling. Feel yourself becoming heavier and heavier. Feel yourself becoming more and more deeply relaxed. You are calm, secure, at peace.

Now it's time to let go of all the tension in your arms and hands. Let's start with your upper arms. As you breathe in, raise your wrists towards your shoulders, and tighten the muscles in your upper arms. Hold that breath and that contraction for just a moment . . . and then gently lower your arms and breathe all the way out. You may feel a warm, burning sensation in your muscles when you tighten them. Feel how relaxing it is to release that tightness and to breathe away all tension. As you curl your upper arms again, tighten the muscles as you breathe in. Breathe in deeply. Now relax your arms and breathe out. Now bring your awareness to your forearms. As you breathe in, curl your hands inwards, as though you are trying to touch the inside of your elbows with your fingertips. Now feel the tension subside as you relax and breathe out.

Again, take a deep breath in, and tighten the muscles in your forearms. Hold it for a moment . . . and then release them. Feel the tension washing away. Now, take another breath in, and tightly clench your fists. When you have finished breathing in, hold for just a few seconds . . . and then release. Notice any feelings of buzzing or throbbing. Your hands are becoming very soft and relaxed. Take another deep breath in, and clench your fists again. Hold for just a few seconds . . . and then release. Let your fingers go limp. Your arms and hands are feeling heavy and relaxed. Take a couple of nice, long, slow breaths now, and just relax. Feel yourself slipping even deeper into a state of complete rest. Now tighten the muscles in your face by squeezing your eyes shut and clenching your lips together. As you do, breathe in fully. Hold it . . . now breathe out, and relax all your facial muscles. Feel your face softening. Once more, breathe in deeply while you scrunch the muscles in your eyes and lips . . . and release.

Now bring your awareness to the muscles in your jaw. Take a deep breath in, then open your mouth as wide as you can. Feel your jaw muscles stretching and tightening. Now exhale and allow your mouth to gently close. Again, fill your lungs with air and then open your mouth wide. Now let your mouth relax, and let your breath flood all the way out. You are now completely relaxed, from the tips of your toes to the top of your head. Just enjoy this feeling as you gently allow yourself to drift into a more and more relaxed state.

✳ The Autogenic Lateral Scan ✳

Lying in your bed, completely comfortable, it's time to sleep, and so you move your awareness to the sole of your left foot. You become aware first of all of your big toe, and then your other toes, which you might be able to distinguish one by one, or maybe you just have a general sense of your other toes, and then you move your awareness back to the sole of your foot, to the top of your foot, to your ankle, to your left shin, not trying to relax, not trying to do anything—just simply being aware and following your attention as it moves, just allowing whatever sensations and feelings you experience to be present. Now move your attention to the calf, the knee, the thigh, your buttock, your hip. And now become aware of the whole of this left leg, from the sole of your foot up to your left hip—just being present in your awareness to a sense of this part of the body. Get a feeling for the space it occupies—its size, its weight, its temperature.

Now move your awareness to your right foot. Feel the sole of your right foot, your right big toe, the other toes, back to the sole again, and then move your awareness to the top of the foot, the ankle, the shin, the calf, the knee, your thigh, your buttock, your hip. And now sense the whole of your right leg, from the sole of your foot up to your right hip. All your awareness is located here. Get a feeling for the space it occupies—its size, its weight, its temperature.

Now your awareness moves to your left thumb. You sense your left thumb and then each of the fingers in your left hand, one by one; the palm of your left hand, the top of your left hand, your wrist, your forearm, your elbow, your upper arm up to the shoulder. And now you sense the whole of your left arm from the tips of your fingers to your shoulder. Get a feeling for the space it occupies—its size, its weight, its temperature.

Now your awareness moves to your right thumb, and then all the fingers on your right hand. You sense the palm of your hand, the top of your hand, your wrist, your forearm, your elbow, your upper arm up to the shoulder. And now you sense the whole of your right arm, from the tips of your fingers to the shoulder. Get a feeling for the space it occupies—its size, its weight, its temperature.

Now move your awareness to the top of your head, to your scalp. You sense your forehead, your temples, the back of your head, your eyes. You can sense your brain within your skull. Your attention moves to your nose, your cheeks, your ears, your mouth, your teeth. You sense your tongue in your mouth, your chin, your jaw, your neck, your throat, your shoulders, the upper part of your back, your chest, the middle part of your back, your stomach, your lower back, your pelvis, your hips, and the base of your spine.

Now you sense the whole of your body, from the top of your head to the base of your spine. Your two arms, from your shoulders to the tips of your fingers, your two legs from your hips to the tips of your toes. You are completely relaxed. Allow yourself to drift into the most delicious sleep, and if you're not already asleep, you can, if you wish, begin again by moving your awareness to your left foot, slowly moving your awareness up your left leg and then your right leg, your left arm and then your right arm, and then down the rest of your body, as you relax more and more, gently drifting.

Step 6

Create Rituals

Into a daybreak that's wondrously clear I rise . . .

—Maya Angelou

*Here, you learn about the importance of creating a
routine for going to sleep and for waking up.*

The idea of sticking to a regular pattern of activity every morning, as soon as you wake up, is popular these days. There are books and online courses a-plenty that encourage you to follow famous names who pin the secret of their success on morning rituals they slavishly follow.

That's what I mean here by ritual: a routine that's really helpful to you. To sleep well, sleep science tells us that you need to develop both a morning and an evening routine. You can make this routine, this ritual, as secular or as spiritual as you like.

If you see your bedroom as your sanctuary, your temple, and if for a third of your waking life you lie in this temple, hoping your consciousness will go to a different level so you can experience sleep and dreams, the invitation here is to develop a ritual for when you go into this temple and for when you leave it—in other words, a conscious deliberate routine that you go through before going to sleep and then in the morning when you wake up.

The value of ritual is that it imbues your activity with meaning. We're not talking about "meaningless ritual" that serves no purpose

96

here, but about a well-thought-out sequence of actions that favours sleep and helps you wind down.

One of the purposes of most kinds of spiritual ritual is to help you access deeper levels of awareness, perhaps even other realms, or spiritual beings that exist in an Otherworld. These are powerful ideas that can align you with inspiring influences, and if this is your thing, then you can apply this reasoning to your morning and evening routines. As noted above, a ritual is essentially a routine action, which is why it can also be understood in a secular sense, as in "Her daily ritual involves an early morning walk and a coffee in the park."

We all have varying preferences when it comes to ritual. At one end of the spectrum, a person might want to do some kind of ceremony every evening, burning incense or lighting a candle, saying prayers, reading spiritual texts, chanting, or singing. At the other end, another person might prefer something much simpler, such as drinking a cup of chamomile tea as a mindful act, or just quietly meditating before getting into bed, allowing their thoughts to settle and opening themselves to the magic and mystery of all that the night can offer. Wherever you are on that spectrum, the idea is that repeated activities help develop neural pathways. Our bodies and brains like routine, which is why even the totally secular and medical approach of CBT-I recommends this.

For many of us, though, our bedtime ritual goes something like this: We start to feel sleepy, since we are going into a dip in our circadian rhythm, so we grab a snack for a quick energy boost and watch the evening news with all its drama, sadness, and conflict. We quickly check our email and social media accounts on our phone or tablet, forgetting its blue light is interfering with our melatonin production. We then shut down the household, do the bathroom routine, and then just as we start moving into the peak of our alertness in our circadian rhythm, having got past the trough, we get into bed and are dismayed once again to find it hard to shift gears and drift off to sleep.

How do you fix this? Firstly, work out when your peaks and troughs are coming. Choose the trough when you want to be drifting into sleep. Work out how long your bedtime routine takes and then set an evening alarm to alert you to when you should start.

To give an example: I calculate that I hit a trough in energy at 10:30pm, but I usually take half an hour doing the whole locking down the house and preparing for bed routine. So I set my alarm for 10pm to remind me to start heading for bed. I used to wait until I had watched the 10pm news, having a snack to keep me going. Once the news ended I began the process, just as I felt overwhelmingly sleepy. Thirty minutes later I'd be lying in bed moving towards the energy peak of my circadian rhythm. Not sensible!

In addition to such a practical routine you might want to add in other components, such as reading inspiring texts or poetry or listening to music before going to bed. Or you might set yourself projects, such as slowly working your way through the works of a particular composer, poet, or spiritual teacher. While you do this, you could be sipping a chamomile tea as an essential oil diffuser gets to work with some relaxing aromatherapy. You could then slip on your ritual socks, because some people find they sleep better if they wear bed socks.

Others find it really helpful to fill in a gratitude journal, or in their minds, as they drift off, they run through three or more things they feel grateful for. Deliberately focusing on gratitude has been scientifically proven to be of value by positive psychology researchers, so don't underestimate the power of these apparently small acts.[1, 2]

We all know the experience of dreaming about what we watched on TV before we went to bed. One of the functions of sleep is to help the brain consolidate memories, and when you experience elements from that program you watched appearing in your dreams (in what are sometimes known as "daytime residue" dreams), you're probably getting a glimpse of this happening.

Why not use this feature of the way sleep and our brains work to develop yourself intellectually and spiritually? Input affects output. Which would you prefer: trashy or even good TV? Or amazing, uplifting stuff, and as you lie in bed, ready to drift off, imagining that you are meeting your inner spiritual guide or teacher, or taking a journey with your power animal, or entering a peaceful clearing in a forest or an extraordinary temple, or reaching a mountain peak with a beautiful vista spread below you? You choose!

Go for whatever you need that will set the right tone for you and help you be open to receiving the gift the night holds for you. Be creative, have fun, develop the idea of this ritual, and see how you can make it suit you. The last thing you want to do is make your winding-down routine a chore that you are only doing because you think it is good for you. The important thing is that your evenings are relaxing and enjoyable. So, for example, if you find that watching a movie or scrolling through Instagram makes you feel good, then that is going to be more important in the long run than whether or not the blue light might affect you.

It's important to know that while our bodies like routine, and it really helps your sleep if you stick to one, it's not helpful to get obsessive about this or any of the prescriptions given in this book (or any other program). When you start to make a change in your life it can help to get a bit obsessive about the details, but once a routine is established, we all need to let our hair down every so often, and sometimes it's just not practical to go to bed at the same time every night. What if we get invited out or the train gets in late? What if we run out of vitamin D or have to sleep in a less-than-ideal bedroom when away from home? Rather than fretting about these things, once we have got our sleep mainly back on track, our natural resilience will cope with variations.

* * *

After a psychedelic journey, it's important to "come down" safely. That's why, in psychedelic therapy, a good deal of attention is paid to ensuring a "soft landing", and that includes integration work with a psychotherapist or skilled facilitator to help you assimilate your experience.

So far, we've spent a lot of time looking at how you can enter into the altered state of sleep as effectively as possible. Now we need to turn our attention to the landing—to how you come back to the everyday world of waking consciousness. The same principles we looked at for creating an evening routine or ritual apply to the morning. Your body responds well to habitual patterns. Sleep experts tell us not to vary our waking times over the weekend; the biological clock, which wakes you up, doesn't know, or care, if it's Sunday.

See if you can create a morning ritual, starting from the very moment you wake up, maybe with feeling grateful for the day that is to come, imagining sunlight flowing through you. In the sleep clinic, we have a particular recording that participants can use as a kind of alarm clock, waking them up to feeling their bodies being filled with energy and light. Some people like to record the dreams they remember as soon as they wake up, as part of their morning ritual.

You can then extend that sense of the morning ritual to whatever you do in the first half hour or so after waking up, whether that's making the bed, doing some exercises or meditation, then moving into the start of your day.

By ritualizing these activities you create a structure to your life. This is likely to help reduce any feelings you might have that your life is chaotic or random and, instead, foster a sense of expectation and determination. You're moving towards being inner-directed rather than outer-directed.

Turn Your Bed into a Gym

An American called Sanford Bennett shot to fame in the early 20th century, becoming known as "The Man who Grew Younger at 50". Twenty years later, he was still famous, now as "The Man who Grew Younger at 70". Photographs and doctors' reports confirm his miraculous apparent reversal of the ageing process. How did he manage to do this?

He found himself getting unwell and aging as he got into his fifties and decided to develop an exercise routine that would rejuvenate him. In a stroke of genius, he developed a method that involved exercising in bed. He wrote:

You know the benefit of exercise; but the general impression is that it means joining a gymnasium, or performing a variety of violent motions at unpleasant hours, which, in time, become distasteful and are finally abandoned. It certainly takes a great amount of courage to get up on a cold morning and go through a series of exercises, which may be directed by a physical instructor or a book upon physical training; in fact, more moral courage than I possess. It occurred to me that as this alternate contraction and relaxation of the muscles must be about all that is necessary, the process could be gone through without mechanical appliances, even while lying in bed or in a recumbent position.[3]

What an interesting idea! Just stay in bed in the morning and build an exercise routine into your morning ritual. Sanford's book *Exercising in Bed* offers a complete program. You start off with simple stretches and end up doing a full routine for an hour each morning.

Add a Brain Exercise from Sophrology or the Silva Method to Your Morning Ritual

You may or may not want to do a Sanford Bennett routine in the morning, but you might like to add an exercise into your morning ritual to develop your consciousness—one that might even improve brain functioning.

The parapsychologist José Silva, whom we met in Step 5, recommends that once you've woken up (and visited the bathroom, if necessary) you lie in bed, close your eyes, and look upwards at a 20-degree angle. Then, at two-second intervals, count backwards from 100 to 1, with eyes still closed. Silva's research showed that this helps your brain enter the alpha state, which is conducive to creative thinking and meditation. José Silva believed that this form of "brain training" could help develop your extrasensory perception (ESP).[4]

Or you could try an exercise developed by Dr. Raymond Abrezol, who very successfully trained the Swiss Olympic Team for a number of years using methods drawn from sophrology. He recommended the following exercise to stimulate brain function:

Close both your eyes, and start by moving your attention to your left eye, and moving your eyeball beneath your closed eyelid, trace the shape of an upward-pointing triangle three times. Now trace a downward-pointing triangle, now a cross, now a circle—three times each. Switch your awareness to your right eye, and repeat—tracing the shape of an upward-pointing triangle, a downward-pointing triangle, a cross, and finally a circle—three times each.

Now move your attention to your left field of vision, and imagine a tree in midwinter, with snow on its branches. No need to strain, just imagine or pretend it's there. Let the image fade. Move your attention to your right field of vision and imagine a tree in midsummer, with fruit on its branches. No need to strain, just imagine or pretend it's there. Let the image fade. Now look straight ahead in your imagination (your eyes are still closed), and see both trees fusing together as one tree. Enjoy this for a moment and then let the image fade.

Breathe in deeply through your nostrils, hold it for a moment, then let it out through your mouth. Tune in to how your body is feeling, just noting whatever sensations you are experiencing in your body.

Finish the exercise by thinking the following affirmation, saying it out loud, or opening your eyes and reading it as you consciously breathe in and out, in whatever way comes most naturally to you, deeply and slowly: "As I finish this exercise, I activate a deep sense of confidence and trust in myself; a feeling of harmony at every level of my being; and I activate the capacity to create a positive future, filled with happiness and wellbeing."[5]

Rather than waking up being problematic—because you feel you haven't had enough sleep or it becoming just part of your life without paying any real attention to it—by making use of the power of ritual, waking up becomes part of a more conscious way of living. It becomes part of the waking-up process in its widest and deepest sense: it helps us to wake up to life as a deeply meaningful and magical experience.

Most sleep programs focus on getting you to sleep. To be complete, they need to focus equally on that fleeting but daily process we go through of landing on the runway of our waking day.

PART TWO

Almost Everything You've Ever Wanted to Know about Sleep

Sleep FAQs & Troubleshooting Guide for a Good Night's Sleep

The integrative approach advocated in this book is holistic. It takes ideas and techniques from mainstream sleep medicine and combines these with approaches derived from alternative healing and spiritual practices.

Sleep medicine offers medication and Cognitive Behavioural Therapy (CBT), which is derived from behavioural psychology and focuses on the way we, as animals, respond to stimuli. While CBT can be very effective, particularly in treating insomnia, some people find it a difficult treatment regime to follow, and prefer the seemingly softer, gentler approach of alternative practices.

You could see the two approaches as exemplifying yin and yang: soft and hard, gentle and tough, non-linear and linear. A combination of both might be just what we need. In this following section we dive into topics related to sleep and its disorders, and where relevant I suggest ideas that come from both perspectives.

Remember you should always consult a medical practitioner when facing health challenges and that the following information should not be treated as a substitute for professional medical advice.

*

*

*

*

*

Are naps a good idea, or should I try to avoid them?

To nap or not to nap, that is the question! I believe it should be taught to young people as a valuable life skill, because it improves our ability to learn and recall information, and may well help maintain emotional stability and our ability to deal with stress.

But when it comes to insomnia, the picture is a little more complicated. In Cognitive Behavioural Therapy for insomnia (CBT-I), it is often discouraged, because the aim is to build up the pressure to sleep as the day progresses towards the evening and napping can take the edge off this. Even so, some CBT-I practitioners are open to the benefits of napping and advise: "A brief nap taken approximately 7–9 hours after rise time can be refreshing and is not likely to disturb nocturnal sleep."

Many people, particularly as they age, find a nap improves how they feel during the remainder of their day, and can even improve the quality of their night-time sleep. And there's no doubt that napping has the potential to improve our performance and even save lives. Studies have shown, for instance, that a 26-minute nap improved the performance of pilots by 34 percent and their alertness by 54 percent.[1]

The only person who can determine whether a nap will help or hinder you is you yourself. So, the message here is to know yourself and to experiment with napping. There are essentially three kinds of naps:

Emergency naps you take when you feel tiredness is threatening your performance, and you grab a nap to recharge. This kind of emergency napping is really important as anyone who's fallen asleep at the wheel, even for a second when they're driving, will know. It's scary! And in fact, there's plenty of evidence to show that not getting enough sleep can be really dangerous for drivers of all kinds, including train and tram drivers, airline pilots, and anyone operating machinery. An inquest into the Croydon tram crash of 2016, which killed seven and injured 51 people, detailed six cases of tram drivers falling asleep at their controls in the six years leading up to that crash. A nap could save your life and other people's lives, too.

Planned napping is when you don't feel sleepy, but you know that you might have to stay up later than usual, or that you've got a long haul ahead of you. And so you deliberately take a nap as a prophylactic, or preventative, measure.

The third kind of napping is **habitual napping**, where you just discover that you function better if you have a daily nap, and you build it into your routine. As people get older, habitual napping becomes more common, as they discover they feel and can work better with a regular nap, often in the afternoon.

So, what is a nap? It's basically a brief dive into light sleep that avoids going into deep sleep. The trick here is to get the timing of your nap right. If you sleep for too long during the day, you enter deep sleep and can actually end up feeling groggy and more tired than before you took your nap.

Have a look at the five stages of sleep explained here. With napping, the trick is to only dive down into light sleep—Stages 1 and 2—waking yourself up before you dive further down into the deeper sleep of Stages 3 to 5:

- **Stage 1: The First Phase of Light Sleep** – This is the "dozing-off phase", when you can easily be woken up. You may experience those funny twitching or jerking movements of your muscles as you drift off.
- **Stage 2: The Second Phase of Light Sleep** – You spend about half your night in this state. Your brain activity slows down and your heart rate and breathing decrease.
- **Stage 3: The First Phase of Deep Sleep** – You hit this about 30 minutes after dozing off. This phase lasts only a few minutes, and then you drop into:

- **Stage 4: The Second Phase of Deep Sleep** – In this phase, your body, tissues, muscles, organs and immune system are restored and repaired. Bed-wetting, night terrors, and sleepwalking occur in this stage of sleep. If you are woken up in this phase you feel groggy and disorientated. The older you get, the less Stage 4 sleep you experience.
- **Stage 5: REM (Rapid Eye Movement) Sleep** – This is when most dreaming occurs, and the stage starts about 75 minutes into your first cycle. With each subsequent cycle, the time spent in REM sleep extends a little, which is why you experience more time dreaming in the morning before you wake up. The total time spent in dreaming adds up to about two hours each night, though you remember only a fraction of this time on awakening. REM sleep is important for our psychological health, our emotional regulation.

If you've tried napping and have found it's made you groggy and grumpy, and perhaps even more tired than before you lay down, the chances are you dropped into deep sleep and then woke up in one of these deep sleep stages of your sleep cycle, which is not a pleasant experience.

Next time, make sure you sleep for just 20 minutes or so. Use a power nap recording for this, such as the one I offer called "Drawing from the Well", available on iTunes or in my Sleep Clinic online course, which leads you into a light sleep and then out again 26 minutes later. Or set an alarm to wake yourself up. Another method you can use, strangely enough, is drinking a coffee. If you drink coffee and then immediately take your nap, it takes about 20 minutes for the caffeine to kick in. And so, as the caffeine kicks in, it wakes you out of your nap.

If you take a nap and find yourself sleeping for longer than about 30 minutes, it's probably better to go on for an hour and a half or so, to get a full cycle of sleep and avoid feeling worse than you did before you began your nap. The best way to train yourself to nap is to use an audio recording that leads you into the nap and out again. Or you could try the little bedside device called the *Morphée*, which uses inspiration from sophrology and mindfulness training to offer you 8-minute or 20-minute naps. An 8-minute nap sounds too short to be of any use, but it can prove surprisingly refreshing. But if you find it easy to drop into a nap, you can simply make sure you have an alarm that wakes you up after no longer than 25 minutes or so.

Probably the best time to take a nap is in the mid-afternoon, when many people tend to experience a dip in energy or feel sleepy. But if you are an insomnia sufferer and also nap during the day, sleep professionals advise you to wean yourself off those naps, so that you build up the pressure to sleep and are therefore more likely to sleep for longer during the night. This can be hard if you've got into the routine of napping, but it's worth training yourself into a new routine if it means you eliminate those restless nights.

A small percentage of people simply never feel good after a nap, regardless of its duration. At whatever time of day they take a nap, for however long, it just doesn't work and it makes them feel worse. If you discover that you're one of these people, just don't nap; instead, lie down if you feel tired during the day, but make sure that you don't sleep. If, however, you find napping refreshes and restores you, and doesn't interfere with your night-time sleeping, then you can happily build napping into your routine.

Work out whether you're the sort of person who needs to nap daily, or whether that need varies, perhaps going in cycles. Advocates of the health benefits of napping say that learning how to success-fully nap helps you build confidence in your ability to fall asleep, which can then translate into less anxiety when you approach your bedtime.

Some people find that they need an afternoon nap during a period when they're feeling particularly low, under a good deal of stress, or during different seasons of the year. In colder countries, people may feel like napping more in the winter. But hot weather can make you sleepy, too, as the popularity of the traditional "siesta" demonstrates. But here again, the siesta has always been considered a short nap of 15–20 minutes, avoiding the problems encountered with dipping into deep sleep if you rest for longer.

In addition to the kind of napping we've been exploring, there's a variation, which is called **micro-napping, micro-sleeping,** or **hypnagogic napping**, after the term *hypnagogia* for the transitional state between waking and sleeping. This sort of napping is what you did if you ever found yourself dropping off for a tiny moment while driving.

In micro-napping, you harness the ability to dive into light sleep for a few seconds to restore and recharge yourself. This is incredibly useful in times of stress, or when you feel you can't even spare the time to have an 8-minute nap. Some people find it their preferred method for recharging themselves during the day, and the technique gained notoriety when the artist Salvador Dali championed it as a method for not only "revivifying one's whole physical and psychic being", as he put it, but also as a technique for dipping into the subconscious to gain artistic inspiration.

Dali said he learned how to micronap from Capuchin monks, and the method he used was to sit in a chair when he felt sleepy, holding a key in one hand. With his arm dangled over a plate beside him on the floor, as he fell asleep the key would fall from his hand, and the clatter caused by it hitting the plate would wake him up. You could try this, or you could try lying on your bed with your arm dangling over the edge grasping any metal object, like a fork or spoon, perhaps using a metal pan rather than a plate, to create a louder noise.

The ability to microsleep can prove really handy in difficult situations. In sophrology, we use a method of running a scan of awareness down our bodies from the count of 1 to 6, which because we have done this many times in sophrology training, can be done very quickly. In only six seconds, you can drop into a state of deep relaxation and then rest and recharge yourself for a few seconds before "coming up" to feel more refreshed and alert. If you're tired while driving, and can't find somewhere to pull in for a full nap, or can't spare the time, you can look for somewhere safe to park for a few minutes and use this technique. It could be a life-saver.

How much sleep do I really need?

The amount of sleep needed varies among individuals. It's a myth that we all need eight hours a night, although eight is the median figure of a range that varies between seven and nine hours. This means that if you only sleep seven hours a night, for example, and you feel fine, there is no point in worrying that you don't get what you believed should be your full quota of eight hours.

The amount you need also changes with age. Broadly speaking, you tend to need less sleep as you get older. Roughly between the ages of 18 and 64 most people need 7–9 hours sleep, while those over 64 usually need slightly less: about 7–8 hours. Since individual sleep needs can vary at any age between 6 and 10 hours, you need to experiment to work out how much you need.

Knowing the average is of limited use, so don't worry about this. Go for what you need individually. Be careful, though, if you think you need very little sleep. A 2022 study that tracked 8,000 people found that those who slept five hours or less around the age of 50 had a 30 percent greater risk of multiple ailments than those who slept seven hours, and shorter sleep at age 50 was also associated with a higher risk of death, mainly linked to the increased risk of chronic disease.[2] Even so, we must always leave room for individual variation. A tiny number of people, for example, have a gene variant that allows them to function on only two hours sleep.

When we sleep through the night we go through a number of cycles that last roughly 90 minutes, with each cycle taking us from light sleep, to deep sleep, and then to REM (Rapid Eye Movement) sleep, which is when we dream the most. We usually need to experience five or six of these cycles each night for optimum wellbeing. If our cycles are of average duration (90 minutes) then this means that we will need between 7.5 and 9 hours of sleep each night. But some people's cycles can last anything from 80 to 120 minutes, so as ever, we need to be mindful of individual variation.

If you're having trouble sleeping, I appreciate it can be hard to know exactly how much you do need, but once your sleep starts to settle, you should be able to determine how much your body actually needs to feel fully rested.

The National Sleep Foundation offers these guidelines:

Age group	Age in years	Recommended hours of sleep per 24 hours
Newborns	0 to 3 months	14 to 17 hours
Infant	4 to 11 months	12 to 15 hours
Toddler	1 to 2 years	11 to 14 hours
Preschool	3 to 5 years	10 to 13 hours
School Age	6 to 12 years	9 to 11 hours
Teen	13 to 18 years	8 to 10 hours
Young Adult	19 to 25 years	7 to 9 hours
Adult	26 to 64 years	7 to 9 hours
Older Adults	Over 65 years	7 to 8 hours

But even these guidelines should be used with caution, as there is a huge variation in individual needs. As an example, if you are over 65 and feel best on 9 hours of sleep, or 6 hours of sleep, go for it!

When should I head for bed?

Identifying your chronotype will give you a good idea of whether you should aim for an early or late night, but a lot will depend on when you need to wake up. If you are a night owl and would do best with a late bedtime, this may be problematic if your work needs you to get up early.

If you can choose when you wake up, then decide what time feels best for you to head for bed, based on knowledge of your chronotype and when works best in your experience. Then fine-tune this with your knowledge of your circadian rhythm.

For example, say that you are a night owl and feel most comfortable going to bed between 11pm and midnight, calculate when you are at your least alert around this time; that is, the trough in your cycle (see page 37 for how to do this), then how long your going-to-bed routine takes (turning things off, doing the bathroom routine, and so on), and work back from that.

Perhaps you find that you are at your least alert in your cycle at 11:30pm and usually take 20 minutes to do the going-to-bed stuff. In this case, remember, or set an alarm, to start the process 30 minutes before you hope to start sleeping. You start at 11pm, take 20 minutes to get in to bed, then over the next 10 minutes you will be sliding towards your least aroused state, creating the best conditions for a successful transition into sleep.

If, however, you have to get up at a set time, it won't really matter what your chronotype is because you have no choice about when you must wake up. Instead, what you need to do is work backwards from this time to calculate when you should start heading for bed.

To do this, first you need to know how much sleep you need each night (see *How much sleep do I really need?* above). Once you have made the calculation, fine-tune it with an understanding of your circadian rhythm.

As an example, if you need to wake up at 7am, and have worked out that you feel best on eight hours of sleep, it will show that you need to go to sleep at 11pm. But it's not quite as simple as that, because in your circadian rhythm 11pm might represent a peak time when you are at your most alert. You will need to make sure that you are in bed in time to catch a trough in your alertness, which may mean you have to go to bed about 45 minutes earlier and simply wake up earlier (see page 37 for further explanation).

Likewise, knowing your circadian rhythm will ensure that you set your wake-up alarm for when you are naturally starting to become more alert. So, for instance, if the calculation of your rhythm shows you are reaching a trough at 7am, it would be better that the alarm woke you 30 minutes earlier, as you start to climb out of the previous trough towards your more alert state.

It's better to wake up when you are coming to a peak and are in light sleep, even if you have not had your full quota, than to carry on sleeping and then try to wake up in the midst of deep sleep, so you feel groggy when you wake up.

Someone told me to drink a cup of warm milk before bedtime. Is this a good idea?

Doctors in the UK used to recommend this, and this is a bit of advice that has been around for generations, but is it an old wives' tale? Although milk has tryptophan in it, which is an amino acid that helps in the production of the sleep hormone melatonin, you would have to drink two gallons of it a night for there to be any noticeable effect.

Even so, some people find a warm bedtime drink comforting, perhaps evoking memories of a childhood routine, or resonating even further back to the experience of breast-feeding. One study carried out in Iran on 68 people in hospital found that warm milk sweetened with honey given at night improved the patients' sleep quality.[3]

In addition, we know that having a "winding down" routine is important, and having a warm drink before bed may have become an integral part of your evening ritual. For this reason, its value may lie not so much in the nature of the drink than in its role in helping you maintain a routine. For some people, though, the fats and sugars ingested may interfere with getting to sleep quickly. But there's certainly no harm in experimenting, and you can always use non-dairy alternatives.

I've been told to get out of bed if I'm not asleep within 15 minutes, but I find this really hard. What should I do?

This is a technique that comes from Cognitive Behavioural Therapy for Insomnia (CBT-I), and it's designed to create a strong association in your mind between sleep and the bed. That's why the CBT-I therapist will also tell you not to read, work, or watch television in bed, and that it's only for sleep or sex.

Making love is a pretty unsleepy and exciting association, so some CBT-I purists believe that it should be banished from the bedroom. Leaving that aside, even though CBT-I has a high success rate, the 15-minute rule can prove to be a major stumbling block for some people. It is hard not to lie in bed worrying that you are going to go over time and wondering how long it's been—even though the therapist will tell you not to watch the clock and just relax.

With the Six-Step Program given in this book, we take a different approach, inviting you to associate the bed and bedroom with ideas of a sanctuary, a place for your nightly spiritual retreat, where the aim is to have a healing, restorative time, which can include, in addition to any sleep that might occur, any kind of spiritual practice or relaxing, or indeed romantic or pleasurable activity. This means that instead of framing the time not spent asleep as a failure, it is reframed as an opportunity to experience the gift of the night—of physical and spiritual nourishment and refreshment.

Is it better to sleep without an alarm?

It usually feels better waking up naturally than being woken by an alarm, and there's a way you can encourage this process. If you've calculated your circadian rhythm to ensure you wake up during light sleep, and if you find yourself waking up naturally at about the time your alarm goes off, reset your alarm for about 10 minutes after you usually wake up, then you can be confident that you have this as a backstop.

If you tend to wake up quite a bit before your alarm, shift your bedtime forward a little. If you find you always sleep through your alarm, do the reverse, and go to bed a little earlier. Experiment with 15-minute increments.

If you find that whatever you do you don't wake up unless you have an alarm, don't worry about this. In the old days your clock would have had two bells above it that made a huge noise, but now smartphones and alarms have a range of sounds, and you can wake up to birdsong or beautiful music.

Should the way I sleep determine what kind of mattress I buy?

Yes. If you generally sleep on your back, you will probably sleep best on a firm to medium-firm mattress. If you weigh around 130 pounds or less, you may well prefer a softer mattress than someone over that weight.

If you usually sleep on your side, sleep expert Dr. Michael J. Breus advises: "Side sleepers put more pressure on their hips and shoulders, which can cause real issues over time if their mattress is too firm—or so old it is no longer supportive. Look for a mattress on the soft to medium-firm side that offers contouring while also providing support."[4]

Stomach sleepers can find it difficult choosing the right kind of mattress: too firm and it feels too hard a surface to lie on, too soft and you sink down too much and that misaligns the spine. What you need is a mattress with zoned support in the midsection.

What if you sleep with someone who has a different preferred sleep position? Going for a medium-firm mattress may suit you both, or if your needs are really different, you could opt for two single mattresses of different kinds, with a topper that makes you less aware of the join.

I often wake up in the middle of the night and take ages to get back to sleep. What should I do?

This experience is called by the medical world "sleep maintenance insomnia"; that is, you can't maintain a full night's sleep. This label suggests there's something wrong with you—that it's abnormal and unhealthy—but this simply isn't the case. The evidence suggests that if you're experiencing this, you may be just as "normal" as your friends who are out cold for the whole night.

A more helpful label for what you're experiencing is "biphasic", "dual", or "segmented" sleep, and both historical and anthropological evidence suggests that this may well have been how our ancestors slept for thousands of years. Research subjects deprived of any cues from the outside world tend to sleep in two phases separated by up to four hours, so it's pretty clear that this is not an abnormal pattern.[5]

The question then arises: *Well okay, but what shall I do about it?* The answer is: anything you like as long as it's not worrying about the fact that you are not falling asleep quickly.

One of the key ideas in this book is that the night offers you a gift of retreat time, a time you can use for spiritual, intellectual, creative, or really any kind of development. So if you want to spend more time meditating, use the time you are awake to do that. If you want to read or do housework, or learn a language or make art, go for it.

It's probably best to avoid exercise, because it's hard to drop back into sleep soon after exertion, and it's not a good idea to watch television, catch up on email, or do social media, because you will be absorbing blue light, even if you are wearing those bright orange glasses that block a good deal of it. Listening to music or an audiobook in bed is an ideal activity, because your body will be resting, and you are more likely to drift off.

If the period you stay awake isn't that long, try using one of the 13 methods suggested in Step 5, and you might find yourself drifting off again quite easily. Even if they don't send you back to sleep, they will be relaxing you and may well act like a soothing meditation, with all the benefits that can bring. The main takeaway is this: if your sleep is biphasic, you don't need to tell yourself you are an insomniac or think there's something wrong with you. There's no problem; there's just a lifestyle adjustment to make.

Ever since my menopause I've found it hard to get a good night's sleep. Advice please!

Disturbed sleep is a major symptom of the menopause, yet, sadly, this often goes unacknowledged, even though one study found 63 percent of menopausal women reported this symptom.[6] Sometimes, doctors will prescribe sleeping pills, but any lengthy use of these is not advised (see pages 41–43), and the perimenopause, which is the whole menopausal transition period, can last as long as a decade or more, although it can also last only a few months or years, with the average time being four years.

Even after the menopause transition, many women find their sleep is compromised or reduced, with 40.5 percent of postmenopausal women in one study sleeping fewer than 7 hours a night.[7] In addition, sleep-disordered breathing and sleep apnea seems to be more common in women after the menopause, and this may be because of weight gain and lowered levels of progesterone, since this hormone affects the respiratory system.

The night sweats or hot flushes common during the menopause often interrupt sleep and are likely due to the changing hormone levels of estrogen and progesterone, which will also interfere in other ways with the sleep cycle. For this reason, hormone replacement therapy (HRT) can be effective in reducing night sweats and improving sleep. Some specialists point out that taking HRT without progesterone may be less effective.

Apart from HRT, the only other recommendation from doctors is CBT-I, and all the suggestions given in this Six-Step Program should apply equally well.

My doctor has offered sleeping pills. Should I take them?

If you find yourself sleeping badly because you're going through a hard time, such as a loss or bereavement, prescription or non-prescription medications might be helpful. Your bout of insomnia will hopefully be temporary, but you should avoid taking them if you are suffering from ongoing insomnia, defined as a chronic condition that has lasted for months or even years. The risk of habituation and potential side effects as a result of taking sleeping pills makes it far preferable to address the problem in other ways, using this program or CBT-I.

It's quite possible to become so dependent upon sleeping pills you are effectively addicted. As soon as you stop taking them, you get what is known as "insomnia rebound", which makes the sleeplessness feel worse than you've ever had it before, so you go back on the pills. In addition, as your tolerance to the medication increases over time, you might find yourself upping the dose. This is a sure sign that you are becoming dependent.

If you are experiencing chronic long-term insomnia for whatever reason, including being perimenopausal, it is not at all advisable to take sleeping pills for an extended period of time (see pages 41–43).

My app/Fitbit is telling me that I'm not getting enough sleep. What should I do?

Don't use it! However sophisticated the gear on your wrist or by the bed is, you need even more sophisticated technology to properly assess your sleep and a sleep specialist to analyze the data.

If you are not getting enough sleep you will know this by how you are feeling and by how hard or easy it is for you to fall asleep and stay asleep; you don't need an app to tell you this. In addition, you risk triggering concern about sleep that can easily grow into worry, which can then start to actually affect your sleep, so that using the app ends up becoming the trigger for developing insomnia. What an irony!

This is why sleep specialists advise you to ditch the apps/fitbit. Remember Viktor Frankl's remark: "Sleep is like a dove which has landed near one's hand and stays there as long as one does not pay any attention to it." It's not quite as simple as that, of course, because if you have insomnia you need to think about how to fix it, but worry and preoccupation with sleep is its enemy, and apps are on the wrong side!

Even though I feel tired, I resist going to bed and stay up late instead. Am I suffering from Revenge Sleep Procrastination?

We've all done it. Our body cries out to go to bed, but we don't follow the urge. Instead, we snack or watch TV. It seems almost perverse, but there's a part of us determined not to "give in" and go to bed.

If this happens occasionally, it's not a problem, but if this is happening often, or even every night, it's worth confronting, since it can result in sleep deprivation, reducing the amount of time your body needs for sleep. Or it can actually cause insomnia.

The behaviour even has a name. It used to be called simply "sleep procrastination", divided into "bedtime procrastination", if you resist going to bed, and "while-in-bed procrastination", if you resist trying to fall asleep once you're in bed; however, more recently—particularly online—the term "revenge sleep procrastination" has become popular.

Why "revenge"? Because the suggestion is that you are taking revenge on the day, which has given you little or no free time. In other words, it's a reaction to a busy modern lifestyle that gets the work/life balance out of whack.

The trouble with this is that the revenge is also attacking in another direction: towards your body. It's as if the mind or ego is rebelling against the limitations the body tries to impose and refuses to surrender to a perceived weakness: the need for sleep. At an unconscious or partly conscious level, there may be a fear of losing control, since as we slip into sleep our conscious mind completely loses its ability to direct and control our awareness. In more serious cases, this fear can lead to *somniphobia*, or "sleep phobia" (see below).

It may be that some people engage in procrastination because they are in fact "owls" attempting to follow a "lark's" schedule, and the issue may be resolved if they simply change their bedtime schedule. For most people, though, it will be harder, since the habit will have become ingrained and will need some work to shift, particularly since the arrival of television, the internet, and social media have made procrastination so much easier.

All the strategies suggested in this book, traditionally referred to as "sleep hygiene", will help, especially those that work with bedtime routines (directly tackling bedtime procrastination) and how to deal with worry (directly tackling while-in-bed procrastination).

In particular, the sophrology exercise detailed on pages 64–66 can be adapted to help program our minds into following a healthier pattern.

My child resists going to sleep.
Every bedtime is a battle. Help!

Sleep procrastination in children is so common it deserves its own entry. Adults act out their resistance through the bedtime or while-in-bed procrastination explained above. A lot of kids resist sleep, too. The three most likely reasons why a child resists bedtime are fear of going to sleep, not wanting to be separated from their parents, and wanting more "quality time" with their parents.

Fear of going to sleep can arise from bad experiences, such as nightmares, sleep paralysis, or sleep terrors. Not wanting to be separated may arise from any number of factors that make a child feel insecure.

The third reason—wanting more quality time with the parents—may arise when a child only experiences direct one-on-one interaction with a parent in the going-to-bed routine. If a parent, for example, spends all day working, seeing their child only briefly or not at all in the morning, and then gets home late or is distracted in the evening by attending to other children and domestic chores, the only quality time this child might have would be "storytime" in bed. No wonder they want to increase this period of quiet intimacy!

If your child is resisting going to bed, see if any of these factors are at play and if you can address them. In addition, apply all the guidelines given in this book, with particular attention to establishing a routine and attending to setting. Depending on the age and the child, you can try reading out one of the scripts given in Step 5. Or you could try *My Little Morphée*, a non-digital, screen-free sleeping aid designed for children aged three to eight years old. Using sophrology and mindfulness, it contains 192 meditative journeys to prepare children for bedtime. See details in *Resources*.

Any advice for pregnant mums?

More than 75 percent of mothers experience insomnia or disturbed sleep during pregnancy. The reasons why are numerous, from the obvious ones of difficulty getting comfortable as the baby grows or as it kicks or moves around, lower back pain, morning sickness, acid reflux, heartburn, or constipation through to changes in hormones and metabolism, pre-birth anxiety, and leg cramps or restless legs syndrome (RLS).

Hormonal changes can cause muscles in the upper airways to relax, leading to sleep apnea. If you or your sleeping partner notices increased snoring, choking, or gasping during the night, you need to get this checked. If apnea is not the issue and your sleep is disturbed, the standard response is to offer all the advice you will find in this book about trying to ensure a good night's rest through taking care of routine, set, and setting. Sometimes advice is offered based on CBT-I, such as to not do anything in the bedroom apart from sleep and sex and to get out of bed if you're not sleeping after a short while.

This is where the approach in this book parts company with CBT-I to invite, instead, a reframing. Rather than treating you as driven by stimulus-response mechanisms that need to forge virtually exclusive links between the bedroom and sleep, this book suggests you see the bedroom as a sanctuary, a place where you change and explore consciousness. Seen in this way, you can allow yourself to stay in bed as long as you like, treating it as your personal retreat space, which you can use for relaxation and spiritual practice.

With pregnancy, this time now includes the miracle of doing all this with another being growing inside you. We know that the mental and emotional state of the mother can influence the baby in the womb, so rather than worrying about not sleeping and getting out of bed if you're still not asleep, it seems far better to use the time listening to music, meditating, reading, and using relaxation routines such as those given in Step 5. By spending time de-stressing by consciously relaxing, you will be affecting not only your wellbeing but the baby's. Sophrology and yoga nidra are both particularly good for this.

You could try gentle stretches or bedtime yoga for pregnancy, as long as your doctor tells you that it is safe for you and the baby. A pregnancy pillow (a variety of kinds and shapes are available) can help if you have back pain or find it hard to get comfortable.

Particularly in the third trimester you might find you wake up hungry in the middle of the night with a rumbling stomach. Make sure you have snacks to hand so you can go back to sleep easily. Hydrate all day, but if you find you wake up frequently to urinate, try minimizing your liquid intake in the hours before bed. The same applies to eating if you get acid reflux: Have your evening meal at least three hours before bed.

Make sure you get the right amount of iron, which is often prescribed for restless legs syndrome, and magnesium, which aids sleep. Finally, apply all the rules for good sleep habits, which you can find in this program and which apply equally to everyone who wants to optimize sleep, whether or not they are pregnant.

Mar de Carlo, author of *Awakening through Sleep: A Transformational and Spiritual Guide for Pregnancy, Adult, and Child Sleep,* has created a training course in holistic sleep therapy that works in particular with pregnant mothers and babies. Her Association of Professional Sleep Consultants lists coaches worldwide who offer this approach, which being holistic includes a full assessment of physical, emotional, and spiritual factors. Stressing the importance of context, de Carlo's approach includes looking at the entire family's sleep needs and challenges as an interrelating system, even when the focus is on helping just one member of the family.

Is it true that certain foods will stimulate melatonin production and help me sleep better?

While drinking alcohol can clearly make you sleepy, there is no food you can eat or juice you can drink that will have a dramatic, or even just mildly noticeable, effect on your alertness. You won't start feeling sleepy straight after eating tart cherries or goji berries, even though they contain tryptophan, an essential dietary amino acid that the body needs to create melatonin.

And it's a myth that people fall asleep after Thanksgiving dinner because of all the tryptophan in the turkey producing melatonin, which then knocks them out. Turkey contains some tryptophan, but no more than chicken or duck, and the most likely cause is overeating in the middle of a day when you have no work to do, and when you might also have some alcohol and end up watching TV on the sofa just when that mid-afternoon dip in energy comes along.

The pathway to melatonin production from what you eat isn't simple. Seeds and nuts, fish, chicken, duck, turkey, eggs, spinach, cheese, and tofu, as well as milk, pineapple, tart cherries, goji berries, oats, bananas, mushrooms, and other foods, contain tryptophan. Once your digestive system has extracted any tryptophan you might have eaten, your liver then converts this into 5-hydroxytryptophan (5-HTP). The 5-HTP in your blood then arrives in your brain via the brain-blood barrier, where it is turned into serotonin, which is then converted into melatonin in the pineal gland.

Tryptophan, 5-HTP, and melatonin supplements are available that claim to help improve your sleep, but they should be considered with caution and expert advice obtained, as sourcing and dosage is critical and side effects can be severe (see the information on microdosing with melatonin on page 129).

Eating foods that contain tryptophan, however, should not be harmful and, although the jury's still not in from a research point of view, it is possible that they might contribute, in the long term, to improving your ability to sleep well by enhancing melatonin production.

Can meditating regularly help my sleep?

Yes! So much so, that a therapy for insomnia called Mindfulness-Based Therapy for Insomnia (MBTI) has been developed, which combines mindfulness meditation with principles and strategies derived from CBT-I.[8,9]

In reality, doing anything that brings more peace and calm into your life will help. So whether it's mindfulness meditation, tai chi, qi gong, yoga, or sophrology, anything that relaxes you and helps you slow down and centre yourself will help calm and regulate your nervous system.

To sleep well you need a calm mind and a relaxed body. Seated meditation, if it's working for you, will help calm your mind, and it should help to relax your body, too, but if you want a more physical relaxation that also includes a meditative component, you might like to explore a form of movement meditation, such as tai chi, qi gong, or yoga, which works more directly on the body.

Or you could try sophrology, which unlike these ancient practices is a modern creation, combining mindfulness techniques with body movement to induce deep relaxation.[10] And for another approach again, involving no body movement but a technique that induces extremely deep relaxation of the body, try yoga nidra.[11]

Alcohol helps get you to sleep, doesn't it?

It's true that alcohol has a sedative effect, but using alcohol regularly to help you get to sleep is fraught with problems. We'll leave aside the issue of immoderate alcohol use—everyone knows the serious consequences of that for physical and mental health. But it's less well known that the overuse of alcohol can result in insomnia, and this is because alcohol messes with sleep quality; in particular, with the proportions of your deep sleep and REM sleep, so you end up not getting enough REM sleep. This leads to daytime tiredness and the risk that, as your body builds a tolerance to alcohol, you drink more to help you sleep, which then perpetuates a vicious cycle.

Small amounts of alcohol, even if they start by getting you to sleep quickly, are likely, according to one study, to decrease your sleep quality by 9.3 percent, moderate amounts by 24 percent, and large amounts by a whopping 39.2 percent.[12]

To begin with, alcohol can help you fall asleep faster and will drop you into deep sleep quite quickly, but this seeming benefit will soon be offset if you start drinking regularly to get to sleep. As you start upping the amount consumed in the evening to counter the body's increasing tolerance, you might well find yourself increasing the amount of caffeine you need to drink the next day to offset the grogginess and tiredness you are feeling because your sleep quality is deteriorating.

You will be effectively self-medicating with socially accepted uppers during the day and downers in the evening, with all the health downsides these can bring. Not a good path to take! The occasional use of alcohol to induce sleepiness might work for you, but make sure you don't get into the habit of drinking in order to get to sleep.

What about cannabis or CBD? Can they help me sleep?

Research shows that both cannabis and CBD can be helpful for sleep.[13] If you're in an area, such as many states in the US, where cannabis is available legally, you're at an advantage: You can consult with your physician and supplier to find the product that best suits your needs. If cannabis has to be sourced under the counter because of where you live, you can probably legally buy CBD (cannabidiol) because it doesn't contain the psychoactive (that is, consciousness-changing) ingredient THC (tetrahydrocannabinol). While as a result you won't get high, studies have shown that CBD seems to reduce anxiety levels and helps people relax. Being relaxed is one of the key conditions for being able to go to sleep easily.

Even if cannabis is illegal in your area, you may be able to source it legally for insomnia through your doctor or an initiative such as Project Twenty21, the largest medical cannabis study in the UK, which is gathering data on the efficacy of cannabis-based medicines for a wide range of conditions.

Cannabis has been shown to shorten the length of time it takes to get to sleep, reducing the time as much as 15 minutes for normal sleepers and up to 30 minutes for those who find it hard to fall asleep. And while it reduces the time you spend in REM sleep, it lengthens the time you spend in deep sleep.

If you want to try cannabis to help you sleep better, you need to know that while its ability to get you to sleep faster is proven, you will most likely dream less, and no one knows if this fundamental change to your sleep pattern, or "sleep architecture", as it is called, is harmful in the long term. The research simply hasn't been done.

One person might say that taking any drug over a long period can't be good, and that we should aim to improve our sleep naturally, without the use of drugs. Another person might take a more pragmatic approach, balancing the need for a solution to sleep difficulties against any concern about possible long-term consequences. One approach would be to consider taking cannabis for a limited period of time while incorporating as much support as possible to promote healthy sleeping, as given in the set, setting, and routine recommendations in this book, with the hope that the cannabis can be withdrawn without the return of insomnia.

A caution, though, about the possible risks of withdrawal: Since REM sleep is reduced when taking cannabis, when you stop you may experience what is known as "REM rebound", lots of vivid dreams. This could be enjoyable and interesting, or it could be disturbing. In addition, some people experience feelings of anxiety or depression when they stop taking cannabis.

When choosing what kind of cannabis to try, it makes sense to go for products you swallow rather than inhale, to eliminate any threat to your lungs. Of the many ingredients that are found within the cannabis plant, two of the most important categories to consider when it comes to inducing sleep are the cannabinoids and terpenes.

Amongst the over 100 different cannabinoids that exist, we know that CBD relieves pain and anxiety and encourages relaxation; CBN (cannabinol) also helps relieve pain and seems to have a sedative and anti-inflammatory effect. THC has also been shown to have sedative effects and help one fall asleep, and since it also seems to improve breathing during sleep, research has already begun to see if it can used to treat patients with obstructive sleep apnea.[14]

Amongst the over 30,000 different terpenes that have been identified, some of these found in cannabis also seem to help sleep. Terpenes are molecules that create smells and tastes and are found in plants: trees and flowers, fruits and vegetables. One of the reasons why forest bathing is now believed to be so beneficial to our health is because we inhale the terpenes exuded by the trees.

Some terpenes found in cannabis can also be found in essential oils and supplements that are said to promote sleep, such as hops, ylang ylang, and lavender.

The most effective cannabis product for you will have a combination of terpenes and cannabinoids that help you nod off quickly and sleep through the night. If you find whatever you have bought is not doing this, you might need a different combination. If you don't want to take cannabis, or you simply can't source it, you might like to try drinking a CBD and terpene cocktail. Although traditionally terpenes are added to aromatherapy blends, they can be added to food or drink, and enterprising companies in the US are now offering cocktails and mocktails that include these ingredients. See the Resources guide for more information.

How about psychedelics? Could they help with my sleep problem?

Using psychedelics as a way of healing is showing tremendous potential, with clear indications that they can help alleviate a number of mental health conditions, including depression, PTSD, alcoholism, and addictions. But could they also help with sleep problems?

So much research into the healing potential of psychedelics is currently being undertaken that no printed summary can remain up to date for long. At the time of writing, very little research has directly explored the topic. Professor of Sleep Physiology Vladyslav V. Vyazovskiy wrote in 2022:

> The possible interaction between sleep regulation and the effects of psychedelic compounds has received very little attention, despite the fact that there are shared mechanisms in the underlying biology, such as serotonin signalling and synaptic plasticity. Sleep is rarely, if ever, considered as a potentially important factor that can affect the response to psychedelics, which is surprising given that sleep is often disrupted in mood disorders.[15,16,17]

Vyazovskiy and his colleagues injected mice with psilocin (the metabolite of psilocybin) and monitored their sleeping patterns. They found that the psilocin delayed the onset of rapid eye movement (REM) sleep and reduced the maintenance of non-rapid eye movement (NREM) sleep for up to three hours after dosing.

In other words, it seemed to play around with sleep architecture (as cannabis and alcohol does in other ways). An earlier 2020 study with just 20 human participants obtained similar results. These are not surprising, and since some antidepressants also reduce REM sleep, there is a slight possibility that the positive influence of psilocybin on depressive symptoms might be partly due to this effect.[18]

But researchers Thomas et al., writing in 2022, feel this is unlikely:

> Given the limited duration of effects, it is unlikely that modulation of REM sleep quantity is a core mechanism of the psychological benefits of psychedelics, although it remains possible that the underlying brain activity of REM sleep is affected in a more subtle way.[19]

The research so far gives no indication that taking psychedelics can help you with any sleep issue you might have, but given that their effects can be so radical, it certainly seems possible that in alleviating other issues, such as depression, stress, or anxiety, symptoms of poor sleep might also be reduced.

How about microdosing?
Could this help with my sleep problem?

Microdosing has become fashionable, with many research projects exploring its potential. Usually the term is used in reference to psychedelics, with people microdosing by taking small doses (often between 1/10th and 1/20th of a normal dose) of psilocybin or LSD. But some people are experimenting with microdosing mescaline cacti, amanita muscaria mushrooms, ayahuasca, DMT, iboga, and cannabis.

The list of benefits claimed for microdosing with psychedelics is considerable. The Microdosing Institute, which offers one of the most comprehensive sources of information on this approach on their website *microdosinginstitute.com,* divides the benefits into mental, emotional, physical, and spiritual.

The spiritual benefits claimed include an increased sense of wonder, belonging, unity, and gratitude for life. The mental benefits include improved concentration and focus, as well as increased creativity and productivity. The emotional benefits include improved mood, self-compassion, better relationships, and a decrease in symptoms of depression. The list of physical benefits starts with improved sleep and continues with more physical energy, enhanced sensory perception, reduced premenstrual syndrome (PMS), and decreased pain levels.

A popular goal for those trying microdosing seems to be to improve sleep, with one study of almost 4,000 microdosers showing 21.5 percent of those taking LSD and 28.8 percent of those taking psilocybin citing improved sleep as a motivation.[20,21,22]

As regards whether microdosing might improve sleep, so far the only evidence for this claim is anecdotal. Some people report that they sleep better, most likely because the microdosing is relaxing them and they are worrying less. With increased feelings of calm, they find it easier to fall asleep and stay asleep, and some people report waking up feeling more rested and energetic in the morning.

It is not yet clear whether many, or perhaps all, of the positive effects of microdosing are the result of the placebo effect, and it might be wiser to try to achieve a calmer state through other means, such as meditation, sophrology, yoga, tai chi, or qi gong, rather than through taking a drug, however small the dose.

If you decide to give microdosing a try, you can find online coaches to guide you. The most sensible advice seems to be: "Start low, and go slow", gradually increasing the dosage until you find the "sweet spot", which stops short of providing any significant alteration of perception, or any other signs of discomfort that would interfere with your daily functioning.

An interesting claim for the benefits of microdosing to improve sleep comes not from the world of psychedelics but from the claim that taking melatonin in tiny amounts can achieve this goal. A number of companies now promote products to help you microdose melatonin. They claim that an optimal dose is 0.2–0.3 mgs, whereas most products offer you 3–10 mgs, which is up to 33 times more than needed.

Their reasoning is that melatonin signals to the bloodstream that the hormonal cascade to begin sleeping should start. In itself, melatonin does not create a soporific effect, as is the case with a sleeping pill or alcohol; it is just responsible for firing the starting pistol. Thus, if you take too much melatonin, it interrupts your sleep because it keeps firing that pistol, sending you back over and over again to the shallow sleep where the sleep cycle begins. As a result, your night is full of strange dreams, and you don't feel rested because you haven't had enough deep sleep.

It is believed that 0.2–0.3mg is the right dose because dose-response effects plateau at 0.3mg, and doses of 0.3mg–0.5mg create blood melatonin levels most similar to those seen in healthy young people. Critically, when people with sleep problems were given either 0.3mg or 3mg of melatonin, the lower dosage generated better sleep, with fewer side effects.[23,24,25]

Someone suggested EMDR could help me sleep. Any good?

If you go online, you can find information and videos on the application of a psychotherapy technique known as EMDR (Eye Movement Desensitization and Reprocessing) for treating insomnia. There's even an app for applying the method to insomnia triggered by PTSD (Post-Traumatic Stress Disorder).

In a nutshell, it seems that EMDR may be a good therapy for treating trauma and stress, and if your insomnia is caused by such factors, then by having EMDR therapy you could be alleviating these issues, and hence your sleep might improve. But it's important to realize that this could apply to any form of psychotherapy that alleviates symptoms of trauma and stress. Often therapists will combine CBT-I techniques with EMDR to address insomnia. As with most psychological therapies, EMDR needs to be delivered by a qualified professional, and it takes time for it to work. It cannot be self-administered or used as a quick fix by following an online video.

The theory behind EMDR is that stressful or traumatic events remain as painful memories that can trigger more stress or even re-traumatization. EMDR aims to help the brain reprocess these memories so that they are no longer so charged, relieving you of much of the emotional impact they might contain.

During an EMDR session you are asked to recall a difficult memory, while you move your eyes from side to side, or hear a sound in each ear alternately, or feel a tap on each hand alternately. This bilateral stimulation seems to help the brain reprocess and desensitize the memory, hence the term "eye movement desensitization and reprocessing". When we process memories in REM sleep our eyes move from side to side, so one possible explanation for the effectiveness of the therapy is that it mimics this particular sleep phenomenon.

EMDR, which has been around for over 30 years now, has been recognized as an appropriate form of psychotherapy for PTSD by the World Health Organization, and clinical trials suggest that the method may also benefit those suffering from depression, anxiety, obsessive-compulsive disorders, severe pain, and potentially even psychotic illnesses.[26,27] Although not enough research has yet been done, preliminary studies suggest a full EMDR therapy course may result in long-term improvements in sleep duration and quality, and it has been used with some success for treating nightmare disorder.[28,29] If you suffer from frequent nightmares or feel stress or trauma may be the root cause of your insomnia, you could consider a course of EMDR therapy.

Can acupuncture, acupressure, or shiatsu help me sleep better?

Anything that improves your sense of wellbeing and helps you relax may also help you sleep better, but it seems that these methods, which are based on the idea of balancing and harmonizing the flow of life force in your body, may be particularly suited to aiding sleep.

A central concept in Traditional Chinese Medicine is that this life energy, known as *qi*, flows along at least 20 pathways through the body called meridians. When the flow of *qi* gets blocked or slowed down along any of these pathways, ill health results.

The job of the healer is to restore a healthy flow of energy throughout the system. This is usually done either with acupuncture, which involves inserting needles along key points in the system, then leaving them, slightly twisting them, or heating them for particular amounts of time before removing them, or it is done with acupressure, which involves firmly pressing these points on the body. Traditional Chinese Medicine practitioners believe there are at least 2,000 of these points, and the World Health Organization proposes recognizing 409 of them.

Although many scientists are sceptical of the very existence of meridians, a range of modalities making use of the idea has evolved over the years, and many people feel they benefit from treatments based on this concept. In addition to acupuncture, shiatsu and various styles of massage also make use of this idea of encouraging healthy energy flow through the meridians, and there is evidence to suggest that they may be helpful in encouraging good sleep.

A meta-analysis of a whole bunch of randomized clinical trials involving a total of almost 4,000 patients showed a beneficial effect on sleep quality of acupuncture compared with no treatment, and real acupressure compared with sham acupressure, and these findings should encourage us to try either of these modalities should we feel drawn to them.[30]

Someone told me about sleep hacking so I can get more things done and even fix my insomnia. Should I get into this?

No. Please don't! Unless you are planning to sail solo around the world, in which case you'll have to dive into the strange world of sleep hacking in order to stay alive on your adventure. In your ordinary day though you don't want to tamper with your natural sleep rhythm.

The idea of sleep hacking is based on the perfectly reasonable concept that we can optimize our lives by doing things differently. Exploring ways in which you can make changes to your diet, lifestyle, or sleep to improve the quality of your life, your performance, cognition, or health is often called "life hacking" or "bio-hacking". The idea of intermittent fasting is one example of a dietary "hack".

Sleep hacking revolves around following a polyphasic sleep schedule. This means deliberately not sleeping in just one block through the night (following a monophasic schedule), nor even in two blocks, as many of us do who find we naturally follow a biphasic schedule, waking in the middle of the night for an extended time before going back to sleep for a second run. Instead, with sleep hacking, you sleep for a series of shorter blocks of time, training yourself to follow a very specific schedule.

Enthusiasts of polyphasic sleep claim (with no scientific support) that such a practice can help with insomnia, eliminate chronic tiredness, and reduce the total amount of time you need to sleep each night. There is a "polyphasic sleep community" online, with courses and discussion groups. There's even an app. One leading website on the topic offers eight kinds of schedule you can experiment with, and a warning about dangerous ones you shouldn't even attempt, such as the Zoidberg, which proposes a rapid series of six 20-minute naps interspersed with 20-minute periods of wakefulness. That way, you get only two hours sleep a night.

And don't even think about the NL4NM20 schedule, an Uberman–Monophasic hybrid. The language gives it away doesn't it?

The Uberman requires six 20-minute naps spaced evenly over 24 hours (as opposed to the Zoidberg, which batches these six close together). The Everyman schedule gives you four hours, rather than two hours, total sleep time, in one three-hour sleep during the night and three 20-minute naps throughout the day. With the Triphasic you can sleep up to five hours in three short phases: after dusk, before dawn, and in the afternoon. Then there are variants: the Dymaxion schedule developed in the 1930s, the Dual-core and Tri-core schedules, invented by the Polyphasic Society, and so on.

If you haven't been put off by the thought of actually following one of these punishing routines, watch a few video diaries of people trying them out. They end up feeling awful, though enthusiasts claim it just takes time—six weeks or so—to adapt. But the science is clear: You are messing with the natural circadian rhythm of your body, and with that comes increased risk of illness and potentially harmful effects on the immune system. You are essentially generating the negative impacts of jet lag or shift work in pursuit of the goal of "optimization".[31]

By getting less sleep than your body needs, you risk all the adverse reactions that sleep deprivation can bring to body and mind, including the increased risk of depression. You may negatively impact your memory too, since long periods of sleep are needed for memory consolidation, and your accident-proneness is likely to increase, too, putting yourself and others at risk.

So why on earth would anyone even contemplate doing this? If you are doing shift or on-call work, you might consider a polyphasic schedule, though matching one with your work demands may well prove challenging. Solo sailors are virtually the only example of people who will simply have to follow one, or develop their own.

For most people drawn to trying out the idea, the appeal is essentially for more life, more wakefulness. Why sleep your way through one-third of your life? Eight hours a night of sleep means that, in 60 years, you'll have been effectively dead to the world for 20 years. Imagine if you only needed to sleep for half that time? You could gain 10 years of life experience! Imagine how much more you could get done! So the arguments go, and appeals to productivity abound, with past geniuses cited as examples of polyphasic sleepers.

Dr. Piotr Wozniak, a specialist in sleep optimization, writes:

As for polyphasic geniuses, the list seems to be getting longer, along with the snowballing myth of the benefits of a 22-hour waking day. Currently, the list includes da Vinci, Edison, Tesla, Churchill, Benjamin Franklin, Thomas Jefferson, and even Bruce Lee. I would not be surprised if Newton and Aristotle joined soon. Perhaps even Jesus might follow up later.[32]

Wozniak continues by debunking these claims. Here's what he discovered about Edison for example:

> The most reliable information I could find about Edison's sleep was his own diary, kept only for a short time while approaching the age of forty. From this diary we can learn a lot about his sleeping habits. He seemed rather obsessed with getting a good night's sleep as his day would often start with notes on the quality of sleep. The better he slept the happier he seemed. That's quite the opposite of what polyphasic proponents claim. Instead of maximizing waking hours, Edison would rather maximize the hours in which he could use his well-refreshed mind. And that's exactly what seems most rational from the point of view of the physiology of sleep, mental hygiene, and productivity.[33]

Apart from the apparently false claims that high-achievers have followed such schedules, and apart from the science that shows us that we mess with the body's natural rhythms and needs at our peril, something problematic is also occurring at a psychological level. The appeals to more productivity and waking awareness through staying up for longer are denying the value of the unconscious—essentially of the gift of the night, of darkness, of not-doing and not-knowing.

The whole thrust of the polyphasic movement evokes the hubris of industrial civilization: of favouring light over darkness, of productivity over stillness and depth, of a denial of the nourishing power of the unconscious, of the temporary ego-dissolution of the night, of letting go. In the appeal to the heroic genius (Churchill and Napoleon are often cited as polyphasic sleepers), we see the lineaments of the "superman" who triumphs over the night. Following his Uberman or Dymaxion schedule, he is twice as productive as you or me, and even seizes years of living from the clutches of the Unconscious, who would show us each night what it means to let go into the darkness.

Leaving aside the extremely rare incidence of people with a genetic mutation that allows them to need only a few hours of sleep a night, the only naturally polyphasic sleepers are babies and animals.[34] Adult humans have evolved to sleep in one or two chunks during the night, and we work against nature to our cost. Trying to sleep like a mouse or a baby is, unsurprisingly, not a path to becoming a superwoman or man.

Can I catch up on lost sleep?

People sometimes refer to lost sleep as your "sleep debt" or "sleep deficit". This is unfortunate terminology because it suggests a simple transaction: a loan or debit that can be repaid. Sleep expert Dr. Michael Breus points this out when he writes: "It's very important that you *don't* think about sleep like a bank account; you can't overdraw the account and then pay it back later."[35] He proposes flipping the idea around to think about using the nights before you might have reduced sleep times to prepare for this eventuality, rather than using the days after in an attempt to recover from any shortfall. If you're able to do this, that's great. Just make sure that you get more sleep in advance of any sleep-threatening event.

But many times you'll lose sleep without knowing that this will happen in advance. Or you might be accumulating a long-term deficit as a result of insomnia or simply because you are on a punishing schedule. You might, for instance, have no symptoms of insomnia and find it easy to go to sleep and stay asleep, but you go to sleep too late or wake up too early, or both, so your body isn't really getting enough rest.

Either way you are affecting your health, and sleep specialists refer to the effects of this by the term "sleep debt", which is simply the difference between the amount of sleep you should be getting and the amount you actually get. Research has found that sometimes the more tired we get the less tired we might feel, so that, over time, we will not notice the fact that we are under-sleeping and our sleep debt will be sneakily accumulating, unbeknownst to us.

The good news is that you can redress this imbalance, but not, unfortunately, with one massive lie-in. The trick, say the experts, is to tack on an hour or two (or whatever you can manage) each night, going to bed as soon as you feel tired in the evening and waking up, ideally, without the aid of an alarm. If you are chronically tired, do this for several months.

To begin with you might find yourself sleeping for 10 hours or more, but that should settle down until you get to the amount you need on a regular basis. Use all the suggestions found in this book regarding set and setting and the need for routine, and this will underpin your efforts with a daily practice and way of living that supports healthy sleep from now on.

I'm on shift work. How can I best adapt to this so I don't feel so sleep-deprived?

If you're on shift work, and it's making you feel bad, it's possible that you have what's known as "shift work sleep disorder" (SWSD). Those diagnosed with this problem may sleep up to four hours fewer each night than the average worker.

With SWSD you may well have insomnia—finding it hard to get to sleep or stay asleep, or both. Your quality of sleep may be poor, and you may wake up feeling unrefreshed. You might have an ongoing sense of always feeling exhausted, and in addition to insomnia and fatigue, symptoms can include reduced performance, a depressed mood, irritability, and difficulties in personal relationships.

In addition to all the potential physical and mental health problems that can come from not sleeping enough, shift work piles on more problems: the potential for accidents, errors, injuries, and fatalities. The disasters of the space shuttles *Challenger* and *Columbia,* which each killed all seven crew members, the running aground and oil spill of the *Exxon Valdez,* and the Manchester tram crash have all been attributed to human fatigue. The nuclear disaster at Chernobyl in what is now Ukraine was also caused, in part, by human fatigue, since the engineers involved had been working for 13 hours or more.

The problem with shift work is that the shift times often run counter to your body's circadian rhythms: Your body wants to sleep when it needs to be awake for the shift, and when its natural rhythm wants it to be awake, you want it to sleep. On to that basic conflict, shift work often throws another wrench into the gears: When you want to sleep it is bright outside, and maybe in the bedroom, too, and there can be more noise during the day where you live than at night (the kids are home for the holidays, for example). And what about social obligations—weddings, birthdays, and so on? Do you have to become some sort of recluse and avoid all these, too?

In order to tackle the basic conflict—the misalignment between your circadian rhythm and the demands being placed upon you— while you cannot completely resolve this misalignment, you can mitigate its worst effects by applying the basic rules of sleep hygiene as given in this book and outlined below. These will also help you cope with the practical obstacles raised at home by shift work.

1   **Set:** If you have to, or want to, do your particular job, there's no value in "railing against the machine". An attitude of acceptance, gratitude, and positivity is far healthier for body, soul, and mind than pointless anger or resistance.

2   **Setting:** Make sure your bedroom fulfils all of the criteria given in Step 4. If you can't make it dark enough, use an eye mask. If you can't make it quiet enough, use earplugs or white or coloured noise.

3   Work out which of the 13 techniques given in Step 5 works best for you, and find a recording of this, if you need one, that you find effective.

4   Work out a schedule that gets you climbing into bed on the downward arc of your 90-minute circadian cycle (see page 36).

5   Keep to a routine, bearing in mind all the information in Step 6, and keep to the same schedule even when not working.

6   Wear dark glasses when you travel home from your shift to stop any sunlight triggering lowered melatonin levels.

7   Avoid drinking caffeine late on your shift, which may affect your ability to sleep when you get home.

8   Avoid the temptation to use alcohol to knock you out when you get home (see why on page 44). And avoid sleeping pills, because

they should only be taken for short-term relief (see page 41).

9 Try short naps or micro-naps during your shift, or just before your night shift. You may, however, find it more difficult to do this successfully, because your body's natural tendency will want to prolong the nap, and once you sleep longer than 25 minutes this can make you feel worse and will probably not be viable at work (see the information on page 106).

Your chronotype (see page 35) may affect how you respond to different shift schedules. Night owls may well find it easier to work evening shifts as opposed to early morning ones, and vice versa for larks. If you've been allocated the "wrong" shift, talk about this with your colleagues and see if you can swap to suit your chronotype better.

If you are on a rotating shift, this can be challenging because you can't bed down a routine for your body, since the changing schedule will keep disrupting that. But what you can do is ask for a clockwise rotation. This means that each new shift will start later than the last one, and it is generally easier to stay up late compared with going to bed earlier with each successive shift.

I fly a lot and the jet lag plays havoc with my sleep. How can I minimize this?

Jet lag is caused mainly by your brain not having sufficient time to adapt its natural sleep responses to synchronize with your destination when you have flown across time zones (usually two or three, as opposed to just one).

It's exacerbated by three other factors: the lack of oxygen and decreased air pressure often found in an aircraft cabin; the dry, warm air in the cabin, which is low in humidity and can cause dehydration; and long periods of remaining seated in the plane. These three factors, combined with the impact of your circadian rhythm being out of sync with your new physical location, can result in you experiencing a variety of symptoms, which all come under the term "jet lag". These symptoms include temporary insomnia for a number of days as you struggle to sleep well, general fatigue, upset stomach, headaches, and mood changes.

Your circadian rhythm, which tells your body when to go to sleep and when to wake up, affects your hormones and your digestion, so it is no wonder that as it struggles to adapt to a different schedule you may experience a range of symptoms.

Children seem less prone to jet lag than adults, and the severity of its effects can vary. Sometimes these seem minimal and wear off after a few days. Sometimes symptoms can drag on for a week or more and make one feel quite miserable. Frequent long-distance fliers are often the ones who try the hardest to overcome the symptoms, particularly if they find them prolonged or debilitating.

Here are the most helpful tips for minimizing jet lag's impact:

1   If you have a choice to get to your destination flying westwards rather than eastwards go for that. As an example, flying from the UK to New Zealand you have a choice of flying westwards via the US or eastwards via the Far East. To minimize jet lag, fly outbound via the US and on the return fly westwards via the Far East.

2   If you're travelling westwards, go to bed later and wake up later for several days before departure. If you're travelling eastwards, go to bed earlier and wake up earlier.

3   A few days before you fly, slowly adjust your meal times to match those at your destination.

4   Spend as much time as you can in the sun or outside in natural light once you arrive at your destination, unless you arrive in the evening, in which case it is better to try to sleep.

5   When you arrive try to stay awake until it's the normal bedtime at your place of arrival.

6   Set your watch to the local time at your destination as soon as you board the plane, and from then onwards, as far as possible, try to stick to the sleep-wake cycle of your destination.

7   Sleep on the plane during the times that coincide with the sleep times of your destination, using, if needed, sleep aids,

such as relaxation audios, earplugs, sleep masks, and even sleeping pills or melatonin (following the advice of your healthcare provider).

8 Stay hydrated throughout the flight to combat the dehydrating air in the cabin.

9 Exercise on the plane as much as you can by pacing, stretching, and squatting. You can exercise even while seated: stretching upward, and tensing and flexing your muscles.

10 Avoid alcohol and caffeine on the plane.

11 Eat less rather than more to lighten the burden on your digestive system, which will need to adapt to a new rhythm.

12 Do breathing exercises to improve oxygenation.

13 If you're good at napping (see pages 106–110), use this skill to keep yourself resourced as you negotiate the flight and the days following your arrival.

14 As with so many things, anxiety and stress just make the symptoms worse and the journey less enjoyable, so use relaxation techniques like the ones described in Step 5, and create a playlist of your favourite and most effective meditations, relaxation routines, and music.

I feel exhausted all the time and sometimes sleep for 11 or more hours a night and still feel tired

If this has been going on for a while, and is not just a temporary experience perhaps related to convalescence or stress, you need to consult a doctor. You might be suffering from what is known as "hypersomnia". Doctors divide hypersomnia into either primary or secondary conditions.

Secondary hypersomnia is caused by an injury or disease, such as sleep apnea, Parkinson's disease, kidney failure, or myotonic dystrophy. It can also be caused by prescription or non-prescription drugs, alcohol abuse, and psychiatric conditions, such as depression. When manifesting in someone with depression, although their hypersomnia is considered secondary, the relationship between the two conditions is often not clear: Is the hypersomnia a result of depression, or vice versa; or more likely, in a complex mutually reinforcing relationship?

Primary hypersomnia is diagnosed when the only symptom is oversleeping. It is not to be confused with "narcolepsy", which is a different condition. With narcolepsy, people fall asleep suddenly and cannot prevent this, whatever the time of day or circumstances. With hypersomnia people can stay awake but will feel extremely tired. With either condition, however, people fall asleep quickly—in under eight minutes on average.

The drugs prescribed to treat hypersomnia are often the same as those used to treat narcolepsy. There is only symptomatic treatment, and no known cure for primary hypersomnia, just as there is no known cause of the illness, which is why it is also called "idiopathic hypersomnia". The dictionary definition of "idiopathic" is: "relating to or denoting any disease or condition which arises spontaneously or for which the cause is unknown."

In addition to any drugs that might be prescribed, treatment for hypersomnia usually involves exercise, an improved diet, spending time in nature, and making sure you get enough sunlight. Since hypersomnia and depression most likely feed each other, tackling both issues in tandem is important.

Is there a link between sleep and depression?

Yes, indeed. Many people experiencing depression either sleep too little or too much; that is, they either experience insomnia or find themselves sleeping excessively and find it difficult to wake up. They often sleep during the day yet still feel tired. This is known as hypersomnia (see above).

A 2008 study found that "about three-quarters of depressed patients have insomnia symptoms, and hypersomnia is present in about 40 percent of young depressed adults and 10 percent of older patients, with a preponderance in females. The symptoms cause huge distress, have a major impact on quality of life, and are a strong risk factor for suicide."[36]

The causal relationship between sleep disturbance and depression is not simply one way: Depression may cause sleep disturbances, but not getting the right sleep might also exacerbate or even trigger any latent depression. To protect against this, the answer is to ensure you get the right amount of sleep. If you can fix your insomnia, one of the results is often improved overall mood, so if you have any tendency to feelings of depression, you might well find that these diminish once you are sleeping well.

As the Sleep Foundation's article on this subject says: "Depression and sleep issues have a bidirectional relationship. This means that poor sleep can contribute to the development of depression and that having depression makes a person more likely to develop sleep issues. This complex relationship can make it challenging to know which came first, sleep issues or depression."[37]

A curious detail is that depressed people often experience more than average REM sleep and less deep sleep. They dream up to three times more than people who don't experience depression, while also getting less of the restorative benefits that deep sleep brings. Equally curious is the fact that some antidepressant medications interfere with sleep patterns and may contribute to insomnia, but since they repress REM sleep, they might actually be helping, in certain instances, by reducing the amount of dreaming. More research is needed, though.

Joe Griffin, a psychologist interested in the anomalous sleep architecture (sleep pattern) of depressives, has developed a theory as to how this is caused, and his theory plays a major role in the treatment of depression offered by therapists trained in the Human Givens and Uncommon Practitioners approaches.[38,39,40]

Griffin's theory is based on the idea that dreams help us discharge unresolved conflicts and emotional difficulties and that since depressives worry, catastrophize, and ruminate a good deal, their dream life becomes more intense as they attempt to discharge the anxieties built up during the day. But the problem then is that the time left for deep sleep is reduced, causing fatigue and a negative feedback loop, as the patient feels worse and worries even more.

Therapists who use Griffin's approach get their patients to reduce the amount of time spent in rumination during the day, encouraging them—often with the use of hypnosis or guided imagery exercises—to use their imaginations in more positive ways, with a view to decreasing the quantity of REM sleep experienced and making way for more deep sleep, with all the benefits that brings.

Someone told me you put on weight if you have insomnia. Is that true? Is there a link between obesity and sleep?

Yes. In a nutshell, you're more likely to have sleep problems if you're overweight (with a BMI of 25 to 29) or obese (with a BMI of 30 or more). Obesity brings with it an increase in the likelihood of suffering from sleep apnea, insomnia, and restless legs syndrome, which is a disorder that interferes with sleep because it manifests as an overpowering urge to move your legs while in bed.

In addition to being overweight having the potential to degrade your quality of sleep, if you don't get enough sleep this can contribute to putting on weight. Put bluntly, insomnia or insufficient sleep can make you fat, or as researchers say in their more polite and cautious way, throwing diabetes and heart disease into the mix: "There is increasing evidence that short sleep duration results in metabolic changes that may contribute to the development of obesity, insulin resistance, diabetes, and cardiovascular disease."[41]

Many of us are drawn to eating not-so-healthy food late at night. We get cravings for fries, ice cream, and pastries just when we should be going to bed. It then becomes a vicious cycle—not getting enough sleep leads to greater calorie consumption, and if we don't get enough REM sleep our bodies burn fewer calories so we put on weight. That in itself affects our nights, we get less good quality sleep, we eat more calories to try to give ourselves some energy, we gain weight, and so it goes on.

If you apply the Six-Step Program given in this book, you should start to sleep better and interrupt this vicious cycle, thereby not only sleeping better but also giving yourself the chance to perhaps lose some weight.

How can I stop frequent nightmares?

Sleep specialists distinguish between bad dreams and nightmares. You sleep through bad dreams, whereas nightmares wake you up and are therefore more likely to interfere with your sleep. Everyone gets nightmares from time to time. But if you're getting them a lot, and this is messing with your sleep and your daytime life, you might be suffering from "nightmare disorder", which seems to affect about 4–8 percent of the population.[42]

The most helpful approach to nightmare disorder is Imagery Rehearsal Therapy (IRT). Using CBT techniques, a therapist offering IRT will teach you how to see nightmares as learned behaviour that can be changed, and will suggest ways of working with your dreams, such as re-scripting your nightmares to have positive endings. You then rehearse these scripted dreams while in a relaxed state during therapy and then on your own as homework.

Nightmares occur during REM sleep. Since we spend more time in REM in the second half of the night, nightmares are more prevalent then, too. They can be caused by certain drugs (including illicit ones) and withdrawal from some medications. People with the following mental health challenges are also more likely to report frequent nightmares: post-traumatic stress disorder (PTSD), depression, general anxiety disorder, bipolar disorder, and schizophrenia. In particular, those with PTSD often report frequent, intense nightmares in which they find themselves reliving traumatic events.[43]

Some nightmares might be caused by overheating of the body in bed, indigestion, or an overload of disturbing imagery seen on television, unresolved emotional conflict, stress, or anxiety. For these latter issues, consider getting professional help from a counsellor or psychotherapist. If you watch a lot of movies and TV that depict violence, try cutting down for a while and see if this makes a difference. The advice given in this book's six-point program (and by all sleep therapists) to allow plenty of time between your last meal and your bedtime should reduce the chances of having nightmares brought on by your digestive system.

There's an old adage that eating cheese just before bedtime leads to nightmares. To determine whether there is any truth in this idea (and no doubt with the hope that they could sell more cheese if they could discredit it), the British Cheese Board carried out a study in which participants ate different types of cheese before bedtime. Of the 200 participants, 75 percent reported sleeping well, and none had nightmares.[44] Most participants also found they could clearly remember their dreams. The study concluded that the essential amino acid in milk (and therefore cheese), tryptophan, was having an effect on the cheese eaters by stabilizing their sleep patterns and reducing stress levels. This is unlikely (see pages 43-44). Our faith in this study might also be shaken, though, by its findings that different cheeses provoked different kinds of dreams: *Cheddar* apparently tended to produce dreams about celebrities, *Red Leicester* brought on nostalgic dreams often related to childhood, *Lancashire* produced work dreams, *Stilton* provoked the most vivid and surreal dreams, while *Cheshire* led to a peaceful, dreamless sleep. Hmmm, perhaps best taken with a pinch of salt? Or perhaps an invitation to experiment with cheeses and a dream diary by your bed?

I get sleep paralysis, and it's very upsetting. What should I do?

Imagine waking up during a nightmare only to find it's carrying on and you can't open your eyes or move your body. This is known as "sleep paralysis". The experience is usually frightening, though a minority of people report blissful experiences. Symptoms include being unable to move or speak, feeling a heavy pressure on the chest, and having difficulty in breathing. Since 90 percent of experiences are associated with fear, often the sufferer feels as if an intruder with malevolent intentions has entered their room or is sitting beside or actually on them.

In the past, and still in certain cultures, these experiences were interpreted as attacks by witches, ghosts, unbaptized babies, or malevolent spirits. Today, certainly from a medical perspective, they are viewed as hallucinations generated by the brain, explained by the fact that during REM sleep the major muscles of our body are paralyzed to prevent ourselves acting out our dreams and harming ourselves or others. In sleep paralysis, we effectively wake up while still dreaming yet are unable to move.

The fact that sleep paralysis can evoke blissful feelings, feelings of flying, or being out of body, and involve intensely real experiences of malevolent beings, makes the topic fascinating for those who want to explore the intersection between neuroscience and a spiritual or alternative understanding of reality. Ideas and research into altered states, non-ordinary reality, and lucid dreaming can all be brought to bear on the subject, as dream researcher Ryan Hurd has done in his book *Sleep Paralysis: A Guide to Hypnagogic Visions and Visitors of the Night.*

Statistics on the prevalence of sleep paralysis vary widely, with some studies finding up to 50 percent of people experiencing at least one episode of sleep paralysis, while other studies find only 8 percent. It has been suggested that bedtime experiences of ghosts or alien abductions could be misinterpretations of the phenomenon. Symptoms appear often in childhood or young adulthood, with episodes occurring more frequently in these populations as they move into their 20s and 30s.

The causes of sleep paralysis are unknown, although higher rates are found in those with sleep apnea. Frequent flyers and shift workers may be at higher risk, and those with anxiety disorders, PTSD, or a history of childhood abuse or other kinds of physical or emotional distress. Certain drugs may also be implicated as triggers for sleep paralysis, including some antimalarials. Finally, having a fever, going through a period of stress or emotional conflict, and sleep deprivation may all create conditions that could trigger an episode.

Some people report that taking a magnesium supplement can help eliminate or reduce the problem;[45] others find that learning how to lucid dream can help them turn a potentially frightening experience into a positive one. Simply learning about the phenomenon (referred to as "psychoeducation") can also reduce levels of anxiety and fear about the experience. It can also help to talk to your sleeping partner about the problem to let them know how to spot when you are having an episode and wake you up. Sleep therapists are likely to offer CBT-I, and in particular, those techniques designed to promote healthy sleeping habits that are covered in this book.

My snoring is ruining our relationship. How can I stop it?

Have a look at Step 4 for advice about dealing with snoring. It's a widespread problem: One poll suggests that two-thirds of US households harbour at least one snorer and that 44 percent of snorers sleep on their own as a result.[46] This solution may be the only way to protect our partner and make sure at least one of you gets a decent night's sleep, but risks losing the intimacy and sense of warmth and connection that comes from sleeping together.

Sleeping pills, alcohol, and smoking all contribute to the problem. Sleeping on your side rather than your back can help; so can losing weight, since being overweight can cause or exacerbate the problem. If the snoring is coming from congestion, blockages, a deviated septum, or narrow airways impeding the flow of air through your nose, then nasal strips or mentholated lozenges might offer some relief, but a more reliable intervention will probably be a nasal dilator inserted in your nostrils.

If the snoring is coming from your tongue partially blocking the back of your throat, then the solution might well be a device you wear in your mouth at night that keeps your lower jaw jutted slightly forward, thereby preventing your tongue from falling so far back. If it is coming from your mouth falling open while you are asleep, then either strips of sticky tape that keep your mouth sealed or a chin strap that stops it falling open may do the trick.

It may take you a while to work out whether it is your nose, tongue, or mouth that is causing the snoring issue, but if none of the above approaches work for you, you might like to try a machine called a Smart Nora, which, as soon as you begin snoring, tips your head sideways.

I frequently wet the bed during the night. What should I do?

In adults, "sleep enuresis", as this phenomenon is called, is likely to have a different origin from juvenile bedwetting. Aggravating factors can include sleep apnea, diabetes, urinary tract infection, anatomical abnormalities, urinary tract calculi, prostate cancer, prostate enlargement, bladder cancer, urinary tract stones, and neurological disorders. Excessive alcohol use, certain medications, hormone imbalances, stress and anxiety, and even genetic factors can all be contributing factors.

As we get older, our bladder muscles tend to get weaker and so we might experience occasional incidents of bedwetting. But if this is occurring frequently, you should consult your doctor. Treatment approaches include the use of bedwetting alarms, surgery, and medication. In addition, the suggestions given in this book should help with improving your sleep and reducing your levels of stress.

Is there a link between ADHD and sleep?

Up to half the number of people diagnosed with ADHD (Attention-Deficit/Hyperactivity Disorder) report having problems sleeping, and it seems that the two issues have a bi-directional relationship, often exacerbating each other. In some cases the diagnosis of ADHD is proved incorrect, with the real problem being a sleep disorder that manifests as symptoms similar to ADHD. For this reason, experts recommend screening patients for sleep problems first, and certainly before prescribing any medication for ADHD.

As children with ADHD go through puberty, they are more likely to find it harder to go to sleep and stay asleep, and they're more likely to have nightmares, too. Sleep problems often lead to daytime fatigue, and both adults and children with ADHD may also be more likely to suffer from anxiety and depression. While some people find the medication given to them for ADHD helps them sleep better, for many the reverse is the case and the medication may actually provoke sleep difficulties.

There is some evidence, however, that all the advice given both in this book and in CBT-I, such as to develop a routine and attend to set and setting, can not only improve sleep but also lessen ADHD symptoms, improve working memory, and quality of life.

Tell me about sleepwalking and sexsomnia

Sleepwalking occurs among relatively few people. Research findings vary, but it's likely that about 5 percent of children and 1.5 percent of adults have experienced the phenomenon.[47] One might think that sleepwalking would occur during REM sleep, when a person is most likely to be dreaming, but in fact, it occurs during Non-REM deep sleep.

The sleepwalker, sometimes open-eyed with a blank or glassy-eyed stare, might engage in any number of activities, including getting dressed, walking around, and interacting with objects in their environment. They might also start urinating nowhere near a toilet or engaging in sexual behaviour on their own or with another person.

With regard to the latter, a whole range of activities can occur, from making sexual noises or movements to sexual aggression or assault. This variant of sleepwalking is known as "sexsomnia" and seems to be up to three times more common in men than women, for whom masturbation is the most common behaviour. It is distinct from engaging in sexual behaviour while half-asleep, in that it is extremely difficult to wake the person up, they have no memory of what occurred once they are awake, and their behaviour may have been unusually aggressive or atypical for them.

Sleepwalking can include not only getting out of bed while still asleep and walking around but also leaving the building and walking or running outside, or even attempting to drive a vehicle.

While most episodes last fewer than 10 minutes and may finish with the person returning to bed and going back to sleep, they can last for up to half an hour. No matter the length of the episode, the person can wake up to find themselves not in bed. Whether they wake up in bed—or confusingly for the sleepwalker, somewhere else—a distinctive feature of sleepwalking (or "somnabulism", as it used to be called) is that the person almost always has no memory of what occurred.

A range of factors that might contribute to sleepwalking has been suggested. These include sleep deprivation as a result of insomnia; the effects of brain injury, alcohol, and certain medications; sleep apnea; and restless legs syndrome. Perhaps the most interesting finding is that genetics and family history seem to be a predisposing factor, with 61 percent of children sleepwalking if both parents are sleepwalkers, 47 percent if one parent is, while only 22 percent of children who sleepwalk have neither parent with a history of the experience.[48]

Although sleepwalking often begins in childhood, some people experience its onset in adulthood. Often no treatment is required, with episodes being rare and involving no danger. In addition, the behaviour diminishes with age. When treatment is felt to be necessary, CBT-I is usually recommended, with particular emphasis on relaxation techniques, which means that the Six-Step Program given in this book should also be effective since it draws on both these sources.

If you have a sleepwalker in the household, make sure their sleeping environment is safe, should they get up and move around. You can install alarm pads or lights to alert you to their movement. When you find them, the best approach is not to attempt to wake them up but instead, to try to quietly lead them back to bed, if necessary using a soothing voice and a gentle guiding hand.

Tell me about parasomnias and exploding head syndrome

The majority of people who suffer from sleep problems are trying to tackle the issue of not getting enough sleep because they find it hard to get to sleep or hard to stay asleep. But a minority of people suffer from more obscure sleep problems, many of which are grouped into a category known as "parasomnias", or "disruptive sleep disorders". These are divided into those that occur during REM sleep and those that occur during Non-REM sleep.

All parasomnias are disturbances to the normal sleep pattern and are almost always experienced as upsetting or disruptive and likely to contribute to or even cause insomnia, except, funnily enough, the rather dramatic and worrisome-sounding parasomnia known as "exploding head syndrome".

The most common parasomnias include sleep paralysis, nightmare disorder, night terrors, sleepwalking, sleeptalking, and sexsomnia (see above). Sleep paralysis occurs when you feel you have woken up but find yourself experiencing a nightmare and are unable to physically move or feel pinned down. Nightmare disorder is diagnosed if you have frequent distressing nightmares. Whereas in sleep paralysis you have terrifying experiences but find you can't move, with night terrors or sleep terrors, as they're also called, you scream and might flail or get out of bed and start shouting and trying to fight off a perceived threat. Sleepwalking involves engaging in physical movement, sometimes for up to half an hour, and sometimes with eyes open. Sleeptalking, which is also known by the rather mellifluous term "somniloquy", involves the person talking, singing, or shouting while asleep, sometimes in normal language, sometimes in gibberish. In sexsomnia, people engage in sexual acts while deeply asleep, having no memory of the behaviour on awakening.

Even more obscure and rarer parasomnias include "sleep-related painful erections" (SRPE), which seriously interfere with getting enough sleep, and "catathrenia", a form of sleep-related breathing disorder distinct from sleep apnea that involves holding your breath and groaning. Unlike snoring, which occurs when you breathe in, with catathrenia you groan on breathing out. Having a partner with this problem is no fun.

Finally, let's look at the parasomnia known as "exploding head syndrome" (EHS), which may affect about 10 percent of the population. With this condition, you hear a loud noise in your head, which might sound like a bang or explosion, while you are falling asleep or waking up. You might sense a flash of light, electrical sensations in your head, or a tingling or feeling of heat in your body just prior to the noise. The experience is usually felt as frightening but not painful. Some people will only experience this once or twice in a lifetime; others report having an isolated series of episodes, or having them occur irregularly every few days, weeks, or months.

The cause of EHS is unknown, though theories abound, including the possibility of minor seizures in the temporal lobe and ear dysfunctions. It's possible that discontinuing the use of antidepressants, PTSD, stress, and anxiety could all trigger EHS, and it seems most likely that EHS is essentially an auditory hallucination, with the good news being that it does not seem to be harmful.

What is somniphobia?

Imagine you don't just resist going to bed, as in sleep procrastination, but are actually terrified of going to sleep, so much so that you develop a phobia. In "somniphobia", you have a dread of going to sleep, and even the thought of this causes anxiety. You probably engage in bedtime procrastination and are sleep deprived through having insomnia. You might leave the lights or the television on when you try to sleep, or even have panic attacks before bedtime. Clearly a very uncomfortable condition, somniphobia is also called "hypnophobia", "clinophobia", or "sleep dread". In a less intense form, it may be termed "sleep anxiety".

This anxiety or dread about going to sleep may have arisen as a result of trauma (particularly if it occurred while you were asleep or at night), and people with PTSD are more likely to develop somniphobia. Sufferers may fear dying in their sleep, a recurrence of nightmares, or sleep paralysis. You're also more likely to develop somniphobia if you've been diagnosed with Generalized Anxiety Disorder (GAD), narcolepsy, panic disorder, sleep apnea, or restless legs syndrome (RLS).

If trauma seems to be the root cause of the condition, eye movement desensitization and reprocessing (EMDR) may be helpful. More generally, treatment for the condition includes CBT and Exposure therapy, which involves encouraging you to confront your fear, allowing yourself to imagine going to sleep, and eventually deliberately choosing to nap. In a more general sense, all the advice given in this book encouraging a good night's rest will be helpful, as will the standard advice on sleep hygiene, as offered in CBT-I.

What is restless legs syndrome?

A common cause of insomnia is Willis-Ekbom disease, more usually known as "restless legs syndrome" (RLS). It manifests as an irresistible urge to move the legs, and this symptom often gets worse in the evening and at night, hence interfering with attempts to go to sleep and stay asleep. In addition to provoking an overwhelming urge to move the legs, RLS can also give you a disturbing feeling of crawling or irritation in your legs. It might occur just occasionally or regularly, and the symptoms might be mild or severe.

For most cases, there is no known cause for this disease of the nervous system, but there may be a genetic component involved since it can run in families. Anaemia or kidney failure can be responsible in some cases. Women are twice as likely to develop the problem, and one in five pregnant women will experience RLS in their last trimester, with the syndrome disappearing after birth in most cases.

Stress, obesity, smoking, caffeine, and alcohol can all exacerbate or trigger the symptoms of RLS, and avoiding these and keeping to a regular sleep routine are advised. After assessment and diagnosis, various medications may be recommended in addition to relaxation, exercise, yoga, tai chi, walking, hot baths, and compresses.

Should I learn how to lucid dream?

In a lucid dream you wake up within your dream and realize that you're dreaming. You might well snap out of it immediately and fully wake up, because it's such an extraordinary experience, but if you're lucky or train yourself, you can keep on dreaming and either just enjoy it or make decisions and change the course of the dream. You could decide to fly, for instance. About half of us will have had at least one experience of lucid dreaming, and about a quarter of us may have them as frequently as monthly. If you suffer from narcolepsy you will be more prone to them.

The experience is an example of "metacognition", an awareness of your awareness, so it's not surprising that researchers have found that people who meditate regularly are more likely to have lucid dreams. Within the Dzogchen tradition of Tibetan Buddhism, the ability to become aware within the dreamworld has been taught for centuries.

Can it be helpful to master the art of lucid dreaming (LD) in our modern world? After all, it sounds so exciting to be able to explore the Otherworld of the dream state with lucidity, and it must open up all sorts of possibilities for learning and spiritual growth. Being able to generate one's own virtual reality experiences without a headset while still asleep is tempting enough, but when you bundle in all those possibilities, too, it's not surprising that there's a whole lucid dreaming industry out there. You can find at least six different machines that promise to increase the likelihood of such dreams, and numerous books, audios, YouTube tutorials, and online courses.

There's even a drug—galantamine, derived from the common snowdrop or other plants—which studies have found to significantly increase the likelihood of lucid dreaming, and thus it has become known as the "lucidity pill".[49] The drug is normally prescribed for Alzheimer's patients but is contraindicated for those suffering from many medical conditions, including asthma. It is marketed in some countries as a supplement, sometimes combined with other ingredients said to help with dream recall, such as Huperzine A. It seems to be well tolerated by most people who use it to encourage lucid dreaming, with any side effects being generally mild, though it can cause insomnia, and in rare cases sleep paralysis.

Apart from the possibility that learning how to lucid dream might help in your personal and spiritual development in a general sense, is there any way in which learning how to do this might be of value for specific issues?

Psychologists have been researching the use of lucid dreaming to help people who experience chronic nightmares and PTSD. For some time now, this technique has been used in conjunction with Imagery Rehearsal Therapy (IRT), in which you consciously imagine different outcomes to the nightmare scenarios you remember. By doing this, and then also learning how to lucid dream, the idea is that you can take charge during a nightmare and deliberately change the storyline. Some success has been reported with this combination of IRT and lucid dream training, but the studies have been small. There is clearly potential here, as there is in treating anxiety in this way, though only anecdotal evidence for this has been gleaned so far.

It's possible, too, that LD might be able to help in physical rehabilitation, with research suggesting that practicing motor skills while in an LD state can improve performance when awake.[50] And then there's the possibility that it can help with problem-solving and enhance creativity. Artists have experimented with visiting an art gallery in their dreams to see if they can glimpse their future artwork before their conscious minds have imagined it. Computer programmers have done the same, training themselves to walk over to monitors in their dreams to read strings of code.[51] There's no end of anecdotal evidence from creatives of inspiration they've received from the dreamworld, and there seems no reason why becoming lucid while dreaming would not help in the awareness and recall of such inspiration.

So there are quite a few good reasons for wanting to explore the experience, but are there any potential downsides?

One of the ways to try triggering an LD involves waking up five hours after you go to bed and staying awake for 30 minutes before trying to get back to sleep; however, this interruption could exacerbate any tendency to insomnia and result in sleep deprivation. There is some research that shows that trying to LD is associated with sleep problems, stress, and depression, but the direction of causality is not clear: People with these issues might be drawn to trying LD to help, or trying may be causing these issues or at least making them worse. On the other hand, some studies show that attempting to LD is linked to improved mental health.[52]

It has been suggested that LD could risk encouraging deliria and hallucinations amongst psychotic patients, and that it might trigger or intensify any feelings of depersonalization or derealization that someone might be having.[53] "Depersonalization" is the sense that you or your body are not real, as if you are observing your experience from outside yourself. "Derealization" is a sense of unreality, as if everything you experience, including people, is not real.

Clinical psychologist Dr. Kristen LaMarca, who offers evidence-based training programs in lucid dreaming informed by mindfulness practices, points out that even though these dissociative states can be severely disturbing, in psychosis or with substance abuse or trauma, otherwise healthy people can sometimes experience depersonalization or derealization (after stressful events or a long session of gaming, for instance) and that these states may be similar to, or overlap with, altered states of consciousness sometimes experienced, or even sought after, in meditative practices.

If, after being aware of any potential downsides, you decide you'd like to try lucid dreaming, I'll summarize here the most common techniques used to induce the state. This is to give you a sense of what is required. If you'd like to work with them, I'd suggest starting with the online course "Mindful Lucid Dreaming" offered by Dr. Kristen LaMarca, mentioned above.

Here in brief are the most commonly practised techniques:

1 **The Wake-Initiated Lucid Dream (WILD) Technique.**
   With this method, you lie down, relax, and try to slide into a hypnagogic hallucination, maintaining your awareness as you

enter the dream state. You try to stay lucid as you slip into a dream.

2   **The Reality Check Method.** Multiple times during the day, ask yourself if you're dreaming, and choose an action, such as looking into a mirror, pinching your nose and trying to breathe while your mouth is closed, or pressing against a solid object. By doing this often, when you find yourself doing this in a dream with a different outcome, you will realize that you are dreaming; for example, you pinch your nose closed and can still breathe, your face is distorted in the mirror, or your hand goes through the solid object.

3   **The Wake-Back-to-Bed (WBTB) Method.** Sleep for five hours, wake up, and stay awake for 30 minutes.

4   **The Mnemonic Induction of Lucid Dreams (MILD) Technique.** Use the WBTB Method, and while you are awake for 30 minutes, focus on your intention to have a lucid dream by repeating the phrase aloud: "The next time I'm dreaming, I will remember that I'm dreaming." You can also imagine yourself in a lucid dream. This technique can also be used at any time, but is probably optimal when applied just before sleep.

5   **The Senses-Initiated Lucid Dream (SILD) Technique.** Use the WBTB Method, and spend the 30 minutes of wakefulness moving your attention between different stimuli, such as sights, sounds, and physical sensations, before falling back to sleep.

6   **Keep a Dream Journal.** Write down your dreams in as much detail as possible.

A study by the University of Adelaide found that the three most promising techniques seem to be the Reality Check Method and WBTB and MILD Techniques.[54] Regular meditation has been found to be positively correlated with LD, and the practice of yoga nidra seems likely to be helpful, too, since it encourages an exploration of that liminal state between sleeping and waking that the WILD technique tries to help you enter with full awareness.

Alternatively, if all this seems like too much work, you could just try using the flickering LED lights and binaural beats of a lucid dream machine. In the long term, a wiser choice would be to use the *Lucid Dreaming, Lucid Living* oracle listed in Resources. It helps you develop the ability to lucid dream and guides you towards integrating that dream life with lucid living while awake in this world.

Afterword

*I slept with my head in an elbow on a summer afternoon
and there I took a sleep lesson.*

–From "Wind Song" by Carl Sandburg

What does the future hold for sleep research and for learning how to sleep better? This book starts with a poem that talks about getting a lesson in sleep while lying beneath a tree. We already know that trees have their own sleep cycles, and research shows that being in contact with trees is good for our health.[1,2]

Thanks to studies carried out primarily in Japan, we know about the benefits of "forest bathing", walking amongst the trees and breathing in the forest air. We now know that essential oils exuded by the trees boost our immune systems.[3] We also know that simply being in contact with trees is beneficial for our mental health, and research in Australia has shown that we are likely to sleep better when trees are in our vicinity.[4,5] Research has already begun to look at whether forest bathing can improve the sleep of menopausal women and cancer patients, and results are encouraging.[6,7] Chinese medicine has known for centuries that mushrooms, which grow in symbiosis with the trees, have gifts to help us sleep. I believe that in the future we will learn even more about how deepening our relationship with trees, with the forest, and with the forest floor with its mycelial network, can deepen our relationship with life itself, enabling us to live longer and sleep better.

Perhaps, as we lie there, our head resting on an elbow beneath the spreading boughs of a wise old tree, inspiration from an ancient text, the *Vijnana Bhairava Tantra*, might come to us, reminding us that "between sleeping and waking, with the gentlest of breaths focused in the forehead," we can "fall into the centre of the heart as we fall asleep." "Thus," as the text promises, we will "fall into freedom as we dream".

How I Developed the Six-Step Program

When I was young, I was fascinated by everything to do with spirituality. What could be more important or exciting than the idea of gaining enlightenment? I studied Buddhism and followed a guru for a while. I also took a degree in psychology and trained in psychotherapy, because I realized that spiritual ideas and practices need grounding in an understanding of how the mind works.

I also had the good fortune to get to know and train with the principal of a college in London who was a historian and a poet. A friend of my father, he was deeply interested in spirituality and had founded a group inspired by the teachings found in the stories and myths of Britain and Ireland as recounted by the ancient bards. His group was called the Order of Bards, Ovates & Druids, and about 30 years ago I began leading this group.[8] This gave me the opportunity to travel the world, talking to people interested in spirituality and eager to experiment with ideas and techniques that some people might consider far out but others find exciting and inspiring, even life-changing.

As I did this, I had plenty of opportunities to become familiar with the technique of leading guided meditations, and I noticed how deeply relaxing and healing they could be. Often listeners would fall asleep, but would still report that the experience was helpful, sometimes transformative. I then produced a set of guided meditations, which you can find online, called "Wild Wisdom Meditations". On hearing them, my German publisher invited me to produce a similar set but this time focused on healing.

Months after agreeing to do this, I had the most extraordinary experience. I was awoken out of my sleep by a very loud voice booming, "Use the Golden Mean!"

My watch said it was 3am. I knew this command was in reference to the healing meditations project, and later that day I researched the Golden Mean, also known as the Golden Ratio or Divine Proportion. I thought it was used only in architecture, but discovered that this simple ratio of 1:1.618 is like a secret formula or algorithm for Creation. You can find it in the human body, in plants, in animals, in seashells—all over the place—and composers have even incorporated it into their music.

That evening I was sitting in our local pub and in walked an old friend, Professor Peter Mobbs, who at that time was Head of Physiology at UCL. I told him of my experience, and that I was thinking of asking some composers to create music that incorporated the ratio for the meditations I had been asked to produce.

He encouraged me, and then said: "You know, you could also engineer the recordings using this ratio."

The next day he emailed technical instructions, which I passed on to Damh the Bard, who was engineering the sound for the project.

I decided to dedicate two of the four tracks on this album, "Sacred Nature", to sleep, since after all, sleep has tremendous healing properties. And I figured that since people often drifted into sleep during parts of my guided meditations, I might as well build on this effect and use it more deliberately.

When the album came out, it started getting enthusiastic reviews, all of them unsolicited and from complete strangers.

They said things like:

I have tried so many sleep meditation tapes, but everything about this one was unexpected . . . it proceeds to a most amazing relaxation exercise, which is based on the spiral shape of the Golden Mean, and is completely, profoundly different from anything else I've ever experienced or taught (I teach meditation). AND IT WORKS!!! Pay attention, insomniacs, IT WORKS! I've almost never made it to the last section, but I know I like it, too. It's a powerfully resonant choral chant that seems to vibrate me into a deep, deep meditative state. Obviously, I recommend this unreservedly.

And:

As someone who's suffered with insomnia for most of my adult life, I was skeptical but willing to give this a try . . . I bought this when it first came out and have used it almost every night since to fall asleep. Out of some 800+ nights, this has worked all but two or three times. Listening to "Healing Sleep" each night has become such a successful part of my night-time routine that I don't even really think of myself as an insomniac any more . . . This has been the single most helpful purchase I've ever made on something to improve my health. To fellow insomniacs I can't recommend this highly enough.[9]

It always feels good if you think you've been of some use to somebody—and now I decided that I should produce more of these recordings. For the next five years, whenever I came up with an idea, or read about a technique that might be helpful, I jotted this down in a notebook entitled "The Stairs to Bedford". This was going to be the title of a collection of meditations dedicated to helping people sleep, based on the phrase "Going up the wooden hill to Bedfordshire", a quaint English expression for going to bed, now long out of use.

During these five years, I also trained as a teacher of two disciplines that turned out to be immensely helpful with this project: one a mind-body training system called sophrology, the other a meditative and restorative technique called yoga nidra.

I became interested in sophrology because it takes its inspiration from the two fields that have always fascinated me, psychology and spirituality, and offers exercises and techniques that address specific problems: anxiety, depression, stress, performance, and so on. And I soon discovered that it is highly effective in treating sleep difficulties.

I use sophrology a great deal. I teach classes in the technique online and have led workshops for organizations such as the Lush cosmetics company, the British Psychological Society, and the Center for Excellence in Public Leadership at George Washington University.

Yoga nidra, like sophrology, only emerged in the 1960s. And again like sophrology, it is actually a hybrid of modern psychology and ancient inspiration. It came into being because the founder of the Bihar School of Yoga, Swami Satyananda, had the inspiration to combine ideas from yoga with techniques taught by Western psychologists interested in the therapeutic benefits of relaxation. The result, which he termed "yoga nidra", guides you into a very deep state that can send you to sleep, and also produces the same benefits and experiences as meditation.

Under the expert guidance of yoga nidra specialists Dr. Unsmore-Tuli and Nirlipta Tuli (the latter also a clinical hypnotherapist with a special interest in sleep), I took a training in how to lead yoga nidra sessions, to complement the education I had already received in sophrology and psychology.

I also took a training course in Cognitive Behavioural Therapy for Insomnia (CBT-I) taught by bio-psychologist Dr. David Lee, author of *Teaching the World to Sleep*—first through the British Psychological Society and then through the organization he has founded, Sleep Unlimited.

More recently, I have joined a team of psychologists and pyscho-therapists working in the newly emerging field of psychedelic therapy. In addition to working in the Psychedelic Practitioner Core Training program of the Synthesis Institute and their retreat team, I have also worked with participants from one of the first clinical trials of psilocybin for treatment-resistant depression, run by Imperial College, London, and I now work with Dr. Rosalind Watts in her ACER psychedelic integration program. Studying in this field gave me the insight that the model used in psychedelic therapy can be usefully applied to sleep therapy.

I have found that the insights and techniques used in all these disciplines can be combined to offer a very powerful set of tools to help you sleep better, and this book, and The Sleep Clinic online course that I've created, is dedicated to exactly this purpose.[10]

Notes

Introduction

1. Swapna Bhaskar, D. Hemavathy, and Shankar Prasad, "Prevalence of Chronic Insomnia in Adult Patients and Its Correlation with Medical Comorbidities", *J Family Med Prim Care*. (Oct–Dec 2016);5(4):780–784, doi: 10.4103/2249-4863.201153. https://www.formulatehealth.com/blog/insomnia-statistics-uk-how-many-people-have-sleep-problems https://www.bbc.co.uk/programmes/articles/10wh9mPTwTT74 0bz74MnY33/the-uk-sleep-census

2. H. Jahrami, A.S. BaHammam, N.L. Bragazzi, Z. Saif, M. Faris, and M.V. Vitiello. "Sleep Problems during the COVID-19 Pandemic by Population: A Systematic Review and Meta-Analysis", *J Clin Sleep Med*. (Feb 1, 2021);17(2):299–313, doi: 10.5664/jcsm.8930. PMID: 33108269; PMCID: PMC7853219. https://www.bbc.com/worklife/article/20210121-the-coronasomnia-phenomenon-keeping-us-from-getting-sleep https://www.bbc.com/news/av/uk-england-40335408

3. S. Royant-Parola, V. Londe, S. Tréhout, and S. Hartley, "The Use of Social Media Modifies Teenagers' Sleep-Related Behavior", *Encephale* (September 2018);44(4):321–328, doi: 10.1016/j.encep.2017.03.009. Epub 2017 Jun 8. https://www.theguardian.com/world/2021/jan/22/children-health-screen-times-covid-crisis-sleep-eyesight-problems-digital-devices https://www.bbc.com/news/health-39140836

4. David R. Lee, *Teaching the World to Sleep: Psychological and Behavioural Assessment and Treatment Strategies for People with*

Sleeping Problems and Insomnia (Abingdon-on-Thames, UK: Routledge, 2018), 119.

5. Lee, *Teaching the World to Sleep*, 98.
6. C.M. Morin, R.R. Bootzin, D.J. Buysse, J.D. Edinger, C.A. Espie, and K.L. Lichtstein, "Psychological and Behavioral Treatment of Insomnia: Update of the Recent Evidence (1998-2004) AASM taskforce review", *Sleep*, 29 (2006): 1398–1414.

Part One

Step 1: What Psychedelic Therapy Can Teach Us

1. Matthew Walker, *Why We Sleep* (New York: Penguin, 2017), 50.
2. *Sleep Med Clin* (March 2015);10(1):85–92, doi: 10.1016/j.jsmc.2014.11.003. Epub 2014 Dec 15. https://jcsm.aasm.org/doi/10.5664/jcsm.6472
3. Niall M. Broomfield and Colin A. Espie, "Initial Insomnia and Paradoxical Intention: An Experimental Investigation of Putative Mechanisms Using Subjective and Actigraphic Measurements of Sleep", *Behavioural and Cognitive Psychotherapy* 31 (2003): 313–24.

Step 2: Tune In

1. Jeremy D. Mercer, BA (Hons), Richard R. Bootzin, Ph.D., and Leon C. Lack, Ph.D., "Insomniacs' Perception of Wake instead of Sleep", *Sleep* 25, No. 5 (2002), 559.
2. Obstructive Sleep Apnoea Toolkit, British Lung Foundation, https://www.blf.org.uk/support-for-you/obstructive-sleep-apnoea-osa/health-care-professionals/commissioning-toolkit
3. Hrayr Attarian, "Paradoxical Insomnia". *Clinical Handbook of Insomnia* (Berlin, Germany: Springer, 2016).

Step 3: Optimize the Body

1. Matthew Walker, *Why We Sleep: The New Science of Sleep and Dreams* (London: Penguin Press, 2017), Chap. 14.
2. H.W. Gordon, "Differential Effects of Addictive Drugs on Sleep and Sleep Stages", *J Addict Res* (OPAST Group),

(2019);3(2):10.33140/JAR.03.02.01, doi: 10.33140/JAR.03.02.01. Epub 2019 Jul 15. PMID: 31403110; PMCID: PMC6688758.

3. M.I. Norrish and K.L. Dwyer, "Preliminary Investigation of the Effect of Peppermint Oil on an Objective Measure of Daytime Sleepiness", *Int J Psychophysiol* (2005), 55(3), 291–8.

4. Mills, Llewellyn et al, "Reduction in caffeine withdrawal after open-label decaffeinated coffee", Journal of Psychopharmacology, January 2023, summarized in the British Psychological Society Research Digest: https://www.bps.org.uk/research-digest/decaf-coffee-reduces-caffeine-withdrawal-even-when-you-know-its-decaf

5. C. Yao, Z. Wang, H. Jiang, et al, "*Ganoderma lucidum* Promotes Sleep through a Gut Microbiota-Dependent and Serotonin-Involved Pathway in Mice", *Sci Rep* 11, 13660 (2021). https://doi.org/10.1038/s41598-021-92913-6

6. P. Batra, A.K. Sharma, and R. Khajuria, "Probing Lingzhi or Reishi Medicinal Mushroom Ganoderma Lucidum (Higher Basidiomycetes): A Bitter Mushroom with Amazing Health Benefits", *Int J Med Mushrooms* (2013);15(2):127–43, doi: 10.1615/intjmedmushr.v15.i2.20. PMID: 23557365.

7. Xiang-Yu Cui, Su-Ying Cui, Juan Zhang, Zi-Jun Wang, Bin Yu, Zhao-Fu Sheng, Xue-Qiong Zhang, and Yong-He Zhang, "Extract of Ganoderma Lucidum Prolongs Sleep Time in Rats", *Journal of Ethnopharmacology* 139, Issue 3 (2012), 796–800, ISSN 0378-8741, https://doi.org/10.1016/j.jep.2011.12.020.

8. Emma J. Wams, DPhil (Ph.D.), Tom Woelders, MSc, Irene Marring, MSc, Laura van Rosmalen, MSc, Domien G. M. Beersma, Ph.D., Marijke C. M. Gordijn, Ph.D., and Roelof A. Hut, Ph.D., "Linking Light Exposure and Subsequent Sleep: A Field Polysomnography Study in Humans", *Sleep* 40 (December 2017), Issue 12, zsx165, https://doi.org/10.1093/sleep/zsx165

9. G. Djokic, P. Vojvodić, D. Korcok, A. Agic, A. Rankovic, V. Djordjevic, A. Vojvodic, T. Vlaskovic-Jovicevic, Z. Peric-Hajzler, D. Matovic, et al, "The Effects of Magnesium-Melatonin-Vitamin B Complex Supplementation in Treatment of Insomnia",

Open Access *Maced J Med Sci.* (August 30, 2019);7(18):3101-3105, doi: 10.3889/oamjms.2019.771. PMID: 31850132; PMCID: PMC6910806.

10. F. Romano, G. Muscogiuri, E. Di Benedetto, V.V. Zhukouskaya, L. Barrea, S. Savastano, A. Colao, and C. Di Somma, "Vitamin D and Sleep Regulation: Is There a Role for Vitamin D?" *Curr Pharm Des* (2020);26(21):2492-2496, doi: 10.2174/13816128266 66200310145935. PMID: 32156230.

11. J. Mah and T. Pitre, "Oral Magnesium Supplementation for Insomnia in Older Adults: A Systematic Review & Meta-Analysis", *BMC Complement Med Ther* (April 17, 2021);21(1):125. doi: 10.1186/s12906-021-03297-z. PMID: 33865376; PMCID: PMC8053283.

12. E.J. Sung and Y. Tochihara, "Effects of Bathing and Hot Footbath on Sleep in Winter", *J Physiol Anthropol Appl Human Sci.* (January 2000);19(1):21–7, doi: 10.2114/jpa.19.21. PMID: 10979246.

13. W.C. Liao, M.J. Chiu, and C.A. Landis, "A Warm Footbath before Bedtime and Sleep in Older Taiwanese with Sleep Disturbance", *Res Nurs Health* (October 2008);31(5):514–28, doi: 10.1002/nur.20283. PMID: 18459154; PMCID: PMC2574895.

14. N. Shinjyo, G. Waddell, and J. Green, "Valerian Root in Treating Sleep Problems and Associated Disorders: A Systematic Review and Meta-Analysis", *J Evid Based Integr Med.* (January–December 2020);25:2515690X20967323, doi: 10.1177/2515690X20967323. PMID: 33086877; PMCID: PMC7585905.

15. C. Stevinson and E. Ernst, "Valerian for Insomnia: A Systematic Review of Randomized Clinical Trials", *Sleep Medicine* 1 (2000): 91–99.

Step 4: Prepare the Setting

1. Rudolf Steiner, *Sleep & Dreams* (Hudson, NY: Steiner Books, 2003).

2. Dalai Lama, *Sleeping, Dreaming, and Dying: An Exploration of Consciousness* (Wisdom Publications, 2002).

3. https://en.wikipedia.org/wiki/NASA_Clean_Air_Study
4. Hekmatmanesh, et al., "Bed orientation and sleep EEG", *Acta Medica International*, (2019), Volume 6, Issue 1: 33-37.

Step 5: Choose Your Medicine

1. Richard R. Bootzin and Michael L. Perlis, "Stimulus Control Therapy", Eds (s): Michael Perlis, Mark Aloia, and Brett Kuhn, ch. 2 in *Practical Resources for the Mental Health Professional, Behavioral Treatments for Sleep Disorders* (Academic Press, 2011), 21–30, ISSN 18730450, ISBN 9780123815224.
2. https://www.sleepfoundation.org/sleep-hypnosis
3. Paul McKenna, *I Can Make You Sleep* (New York: Bantam, 2009).
4. R. Rouw and M. Erfanian, "A Large-Scale Study of Misophonia", *J Clin Psychol.* (March 2018);74(3):453–479. doi: 10.1002/jclp.22500. Epub 2017 May 31. PMID: 28561277.
5. N.V. Reddy and A.B. Mohabbat, "Autonomous Sensory Meridian Response: Your Patients Already Know, Do You?" *Cleve Clin J Med.* (November 23, 2020);87(12):751–754, doi: 10.3949/ccjm.87a.20005. PMID: 33229391.

Step 6: Create Rituals

1. M.E. Seligman, T.A. Steen, N. Park, and C. Peterson, "Positive Psychology Progress: Empirical Validation of Interventions." *American Psychologist* (2005); 60(5), 410.
2. R.A. Emmons and R. Stern, "Gratitude as a Psychotherapeutic Intervention", *Journal of Clinical Psychology* (2013); 69(8), 846–855.
3. Sanford Bennet, *Exercising in Bed* (Ireland: Hardpress Publishing, 2014).
4. José Silva, *The Silva Mind Control Method* (New York: Gallery Books, 2022).
5. Raymond Abrezol, *Vaincre par la sophrologie: Exploiter son potentiel physique et psychologique* (Paris, France: Editions Lanore, 2007).

Part Two
Sleep FAQs & Troubleshooting Guide
for a Good Night's Sleep

1. https://www.nasa.gov/vision/space/livinginspace/03jun_naps.html
2. S. Sabia, A. Dugravot, D. Léger, C. Ben Hassen, M. Kivimaki, et al. "Association of Sleep Duration at Age 50, 60, and 70 years with Risk of Multimorbidity in the UK: 25-Year Follow-Up of the Whitehall II Cohort Study", *PLOS Medicine* 19 (2022) (10): e1004109. https://doi.org/10.1371/journal.pmed.
3. A. Fakhr-Movahedi, M. Mirmohammadkhani, and H. Ramezani, "Effect of Milk-Honey Mixture on the Sleep Quality of Coronary Patients: A Clinical Trial Study", *Clin Nutr* ESPEN (December 2018);28:132–135, doi: 10.1016/j.clnesp.2018.08.015. Epub 2018 Sep 10. PMID: 30390870.
4. Dr. Michael Breus, thesleepdoctor.com
5. T.A. Wehr, "In Short Photoperiods, Human Sleep Is Biphasic", *J Sleep Res.* (June 1992);1(2):103–107, doi: 10.1111/j.1365-2869.1992.tb00019.x. PMID: 10607034.
6. H. Hachul, A.G. Bezerra, and M.L. Andersen, "Insomnia and Menopause. In H. Attarian, (ed) *Clinical Handbook of Insomnia: Current Clinical Neurology* (Springer, Cham., 2017) https://doi.org/10.1007/978-3-319-41400-3_10
7. P. Proserpio, S. Marra, C. Campana, E.C. Agostoni, L. Palagini, L. Nobili, and R.E. Nappi, "Insomnia and Menopause: A Narrative Review on Mechanisms and Treatments", *Climacteric* (December 2020);23(6):539–549, doi: 10.1080/13697137.2020.1799973. Epub 2020 Sep 3. PMID: 32880197.
8. D.S. Black, G.A. O'Reilly, R. Olmstead, E.C. Breen, and M.R. Irwin, "Mindfulness Meditation and Improvement in Sleep Quality and Daytime Impairment Among Older Adults With Sleep Disturbances: A Randomized Clinical Trial", *JAMA Intern Med.* (2015);175(4):494–501, doi:10.1001/jamainternmed.2014.8081
9. N. Caycedo Desprez, K. van Rangelrooij, M. Fernández García, J. Fernández Rovira, M. Molina Ayala, R. Solans Buxeda, and

A. Bulbena Vilarrasa, "Efficacité du programme 'Mieux dormir & sophrologie' chez les patients d'un centre médical de soins primaires souffrant d'insomnie chronique. Une étude prospective randomisée et contrôlée", *Hegel* 3 (2020), 201–209. https://doi.org/10.3917/heg.103.0201

10. K. Datta, M. Tripathi, M. Verma, D. Masiwal, H.N. Mallick. "Yoga Nidra Practice Shows Improvement in Sleep in Patients with Chronic Insomnia: A Randomized Controlled Trial", *Natl Med J India* (May–June 2021);34(3):143–150. doi: 10.25259/NMJI_63_19. PMID: 34825538.

11. J.C. Ong, R. Manber, Z. Segal, Y. Xia, S. Shapiro, and J.K. Wyatt, "A Randomized Controlled Trial of Mindfulness Meditation for Chronic Insomnia", *Sleep* (September 1, 2014);37(9):1553-63, doi: 10.5665/sleep.4010. PMID: 25142566; PMCID: PMC4153063.

12. J. Pietilä, E. Helander, I. Korhonen, T. Myllymäki, U.M. Kujala, H. Lindholm, "Acute Effect of Alcohol Intake on Cardiovascular Autonomic Regulation during the First Hours of Sleep in a Large Real-World Sample of Finnish Employees: Observational Study", *JMIR Ment Health* (March 16, 2018);5(1):e23, doi: 10.2196/mental.9519. PMID: 29549064; PMCID: PMC5878366.

13. K. A. Babson, J. Sottile, D. Morabito, "Cannabis, Cannabinoids, and Sleep: A Review of the Literature," *Curr Psychiatry Rep.* (April 2017);19(4):23, doi: 10.1007/s11920-017-0775-9. PMID: 28349316.

14. Bhrati Prasad, Miodrag Radulovacki, and David Carley, "Proof of Concept Trial of Dronabinol in Obstructive Sleep Apnea", *Frontiers in Psychiatry* 4 (2013), doi: 10.3389/fpsyt.2013.00001.

15. C.W. Thomas, C. Blanco-Duque, B.J. Bréant, et al, "Psilocin Acutely Alters Sleep-Wake Architecture and Cortical Brain Activity in Laboratory Mice", *Transl Psychiatry* 12 (2022), 77. https://doi.org/10.1038/s41398-022-01846-9

16. https://areterecovery.com/psychedelic-drugs-affect-sleep/

17. J.N. Muzio, H.P. Roffwarg, and E. Kaufman, "Alterations in the Nocturnal Sleep Cycle Resulting from LSD", *Electroencephalography and Clinical Neurophysiology* 21 (1966) (4), 313–324. https://doi.org/10.1016/0013-4694(66)90037-X

18. D. Dudysová, K. Janků, M. Šmotek, E. Saifutdinova, J. Kopřivová, J. Bušková, et al, "The Effects of Daytime Psilocybin Administration on Sleep: Implications for Antidepressant Action", *Front Pharmacol* (2020);11.

19. J.M. Rootman, P. Kryskow, K. Harvey, et al, "Adults Who Microdose Psychedelics Report Health Related Motivations and Lower Levels of Anxiety and Depression Compared to Non-Microdosers", *Sci Rep* 11 (2021), 22479. https://doi.org/10.1038/s41598-021-01811-4

20. J.M. Rootman, M. Kiraga, P. Kryskow, et al, "Psilocybin Microdosers Demonstrate Greater Observed Improvements in Mood and Mental Health at One Month Relative to Non-Microdosing Controls", *Sci Rep* 12 (2022), 11091. https://doi.org/10.1038/s41598-022-14512-3

21. Muzio, Roffwarg, and Kaufman, "Alterations in the Nocturnal Sleep Cycle Resulting from LSD", 313–324. https://doi.org/10.1016/0013-4694(66)90037-X

22. B. Masha, *Microdosing with Amanita Muscaria* (New York: Simon and Schuster, 2022).

23. Irina V. Zhdanova, Richard J. Wurtman, Meredith M. Regan, Judith A. Taylor, Jian Ping Shi, and Ojingwa U. Leclair, "Melatonin Treatment for Age-Related Insomnia", *The Journal of Clinical Endocrinology & Metabolism* 86 (1 October, 2001), Issue 10, 4727–4730. https://doi.org/10.1210/jcem.86.10.7901

24. A. Brzezinski, M.G. Vangel, R.J. Wurtman, G. Norrie, I. Zhdanova, A. Ben-Shushan, and I. Ford, "Effects of Exogenous Melatonin on Sleep: A Meta-Analysis", *Sleep Med Rev* (February 2005);9(1):41–50, doi: 10.1016/j.smrv.2004.06.004. PMID: 15649737.

25. E.M. Vural, B.C. van Munster, and S.E. de Rooij, "Optimal Dosages for Melatonin Supplementation Therapy in Older Adults: A Systematic Review of Current Literature", *Drugs Aging* (June 2014);31(6):441–51, doi: 10.1007/s40266-014-0178-0. PMID: 24802882.

26. G. Castelnuovo, I. Fernandez, and B.L. Amann, "Editorial: Present and Future of EMDR in Clinical Psychology and

Psychotherapy", *Front. Psychol.* (2019) 10:2185, doi: 10.3389/fpsyg.2019.02185.

27. A. Valiente-Gómez, A. Moreno-Alcázar, D. Treen, C. Cedrón, F. Colom, V. Pérez, and B.L. Amann, "EMDR beyond PTSD: A Systematic Literature Review", *Front Psychol.* (September 26, 2017);8:1668, doi: 10.3389/fpsyg.2017.01668. PMID: 29018388; PMCID: PMC5623122.

28. M. R. Raboni, F.F.D. Alonso, S. Tufik, and D. Suchecki, "Improvement of Mood and Sleep Alterations in Posttraumatic Stress Disorder Patients by Eye Movement Desensitization and Reprocessing, *Front. Behav. Neu*rosci 8 (2014).

29. N. Ghanbari, N.A. Afrasiabifar, and R.Z. Cooper, "The Effect of EMDR Versus Guided Imagery on Insomnia Severity in Patients With Rheumatoid Arthritis", *Journal of EMDR Practice and Research* 13 (2019) (1): 2–9, doi:10.1891/1933-3196.13.1.2.

30. H. Cao, X. Pan, H. Li, and J. Liu, "Acupuncture for Treatment of Insomnia: A Systematic Review of Randomized Controlled Trials", *J Altern Complement Med.* (November, 2009);15(11):1171–86, doi: 10.1089/acm.2009.0041. PMID: 19922248; PMCID: PMC3156618.

31. M.D. Weaver, T.L. Sletten, R.G. Foster, D. Gozal, E.B. Klerman, S.M.W. Rajaratnam, T. Roenneberg, J.S. Takahashi, F.W. Turek, M.V. Vitiello, et al, "Adverse Impact of Polyphasic Sleep Patterns in Humans: Report of the National Sleep Foundation Sleep Timing and Variability Consensus Panel", *Sleep Health* (June 2021);7(3):293–302, doi: 10.1016/j.sleh.2021.02.009. Epub 2021 Mar 29. PMID: 33795195.

32. https://supermemo.guru/wiki/Science_of_sleep

33. https://www.scientificamerican.com/article/genetic-mutation-sleep-less/

34. https://thesleepdoctor.com/sleep-deprivation/sleep-debt/

35. D. Nutt, S. Wilson, and L. Paterson, "Sleep Disorders as Core Symptoms of Depression", *Dialogues Clin Neurosci* (2008);10(3): 329–36, doi: 10.31887/DCNS.2008.10.3/dnutt. PMID: 18979946; PMCID: PMC3181883.

36. https://www.sleepfoundation.org/mental-health/depression-and-sleep

37. https://en.wikipedia.org/wiki/Expectation_fulfilment_theory_of_dreaming

38. http://www.unifiedpsychotherapyproject.org/psychotherapedia/index.php/Human_Givens#Expectation_fulfilment_theory_of_dreaming_and_its_link_to_Human_Givens_therapy

39. Joe Griffin and IvanTyrrell, *Why We Dream: The Definitive Answer* (Hailsham, UK: Human Givens Publishing, 2014).

40. S. Taheri. "The Link between Short Sleep Duration and Obesity: We Should Recommend More Sleep to Prevent Obesity", *Arch Dis Child.* (November 2006); 91(11):88–4, doi: 10.1136/adc.2005.093013. PMID: 17056861; PMCID: PMC2082964.

41. https://www.sleepfoundation.org/nightmares

42. R. Levin and T.A. Nielsen, "Disturbed Dreaming, Posttraumatic Stress Disorder, and Affect Distress: A Review and Neurocognitive Model", *Psychological Bulletin, 133* (2007) (3), 482–528.

43. https://www.nature.com/scitable/blog/mind-read/sweet_dreams_are_made_of/

44. L. Popoviciu, D. Delast-Popoviciu, R. Delast-Popoviciu, I. Bagathai, G. Bicher, C. Buksa, S. Covaciu, and E. Szalay, "Parasomnias (Non-Epileptic Nocturnal Episodic Manifestations) in Patients with Magnesium Deficiency", *Rom J Neurol Psychiatry* (January–March 1990);28(1):19–24. PMID: 2242333.

45. https://www.multivu.com/players/English/8965351-mute-snoring-harris-poll/

46. H.M. Stallman and M. Kohler, "Prevalence of Sleepwalking: A Systematic Review and Meta-Analysis", *PLoS One* (November 10, 2016);11(11):e0164769, doi: 10.1371/journal.pone.0164769. PMID: 27832078; PMCID: PMC5104520.

47. C. Hublin, J. Kaprio, M. Partinen, K. Heikkilä, M. Koskenvuo, "Prevalence and Genetics of Sleepwalking: A Population-Based Twin Study", *Neurology* (January 1997);48(1):177–81, doi: 10.1212/wnl.48.1.177. PMID: 9008515.

48. S. LaBerge, K. LaMarca, and B. Baird, "Pre-Sleep Treatment with Galantamine Stimulates Lucid Dreaming: A Double-Blind, Placebo-Controlled, Crossover Study", *PLoS One* (August 8, 2018);13(8):e0201246. doi: 10.1371/journal.pone.0201246. PMID: 30089135; PMCID: PMC6082533.

49. Sérgio A. Mota-Rolim and John F. Araujo, "Neurobiology and Clinical Implications of Lucid Dreaming", *Medical Hypotheses* 81 (2013), Issue 5, 751–756, ISSN 0306-9877, https://doi.org/10.1016/j.mehy.2013.04.049.

50. D. Barrett, "Dreams and Creative Problem-Solving", *Ann N Y Acad Sci* (October 2017);1406(1):64–67, doi: 10.1111/nyas.13412. Epub 2017 Jun 22. PMID: 28640937.

51. L. Aviram and N. Soffer-Dudek, "Lucid Dreaming: Intensity, But Not Frequency, Is Inversely Related to Psychopathology", *Front Psychol* (March 22, 2018);9:384, doi: 10.3389/fpsyg.2018.00384. PMID: 29623062; PMCID: PMC5875414.

52. B. Holzinger, B. Saletu, and G. Klösch, "Cognitions in Sleep: Lucid Dreaming as an Intervention for Nightmares in Patients With Posttraumatic Stress Disorder", *Front Psychol.* (August 21, 2020);11:1826, doi: 10.3389/fpsyg.2020.01826. PMID: 32973600; PMCID: PMC7471655.

53. N.B. Mota, A. Resende, S.A. Mota-Rolim, M. Copelli, S. Ribeiro, "Psychosis and the Control of Lucid Dreaming", *Front Psychol* (March 9, 2016);7:294, doi: 10.3389/fpsyg.2016.00294. PMID: 27014118; PMCID: PMC4783408.

54. D.J. Aspy, P. Delfabbro, M. Proeve, and P. Mohr, "Reality Testing and the Mnemonic Induction of Lucid Dreams: Findings from the National Australian Lucid Dream Induction Study", *Dreaming* (2017)27(3), 206–231. https://doi.org/10.1037/drm0000059

Afterword

1. Eetu Puttonen, Christian Briese, Gottfried Mandlburger, Martin Wieser, Martin Pfennigbauer, András Zlinszky, and Norbert Pfeifer, "Quantification of Overnight Movement of Birch (Betula

pendula) Branches and Foliage with Short Interval Terrestrial Laser Scanning", *Frontiers in Plant Science* 7 (2016).

2. O. Kardan, P. Gozdyra, B. Misic. et al, "Neighborhood Greenspace and Health in a Large Urban Center", *Sci Rep* 5 (2015), 11610. https://doi.org/10.1038/srep11610
https://www.hsph.harvard.edu/news/hsph-in-the-news/the-health-benefits-of-trees/

3. Q. Li, "Effect of Forest Bathing Trips on Human Immune Function", *Environ Health Prev Med.* (January, 2010);15(1):9–17, doi: 10.1007/s12199-008-0068-3. PMID: 19568839; PMCID: PMC2793341.

4. M.R. Marselle, D.E. Bowler, J. Watzema, et al, "Urban Street Tree Biodiversity and Antidepressant Prescriptions", *Sci Rep* 10 (2020); 22445. https://doi.org/10.1038/s41598-020-79924-5

5. Thomas Astell-Burt and Xiaoqi Feng, *SSM - Population Health* 10 (2020).

6. H. Kim, J. Kim, H.J. Ju, B.J. Jang, T.K. Wang, and Y.I. Kim, "Effect of Forest Therapy for Menopausal Women with Insomnia", *Int J Environ Res Public Health* (Septeber 9, 2020);17(18):6548, doi: 10.3390/ijerph17186548. PMID: 32916805; PMCID: PMC7558331.

7. Q. Li, K. Morimoto, A. Nakadai, H. Inagaki, M. Katsumata, T. Shimizu, Y. Hirata, K. Hirata, H. Suzuki, Y. Miyazaki, et al, "Forest Bathing Enhances Human Natural Killer Activity and Expression of Anti-Cancer Proteins", *Int J Immunopathol Pharmacol* April–June 2007);20(2 Suppl 2):3–8, doi: 10.1177/03946320070200S202. PMID: 17903349.

How I Developed the Six-Step Program

1. The Order of Bards Ovates & Druids website is druidry.org

2. The collections of *Wild Wisdom Meditations* and *Sacred Nature Meditations*, which includes the "Healing Sleep" track, are available from iTunes and Amazon.

3. My Sleep Clinic course is available at: philipcarr-gomm.com/courses

Resources

"Knowledge is Power" said Francis Bacon, and research has shown that when people gain more knowledge about sleep, the quality of their sleep can improve. This could be because when we understand something, we feel more empowered, more in control, so we are less likely to feel that we are victims of something beyond our understanding. The topic of sleep—how it works, the history of its research, and so on—is fascinating, as revealed in the books and films listed here.

Online Tests

You might like to begin your exploration of this topic by taking some online tests to learn more about your own sleep profile.

Sleep Apnea. First, make sure that you don't suffer from sleep apnea (also spelled "apnoea" in the UK). The main symptoms of this condition are: your breathing stops and starts while you sleep; you make gasping, snorting, or choking noises while you sleep; you always feel very tired during the day. See your doctor or look online for home tests as a first step.

Chronotype. Find out your "chronotype", which will help you work out when you sleep best. Sleep specialist Dr. Michael Breus offers definitions of four chronotypes (Lions, Bears, Wolves, and Dolphins) and an online test. Visit *chronoquiz.com*

Programs to Help You Sleep Better

The Sleep Clinic. For an online program that works with the integrative approach given in this book, combining sleep science with alternative and spiritually based techniques and accessible online with specially designed audio tracks and accompanying films, visit *thesleepclinic.org.uk*

Yoga Nidra. The Yoga Nidra Network offers an excellent online course that provides those suffering from insomnia with an understanding of how sleep works and of how to sleep well, as well as the basics they need to apply the practice of yoga nidra therapeutically to their condition. It is presented by clinical hypnotherapist Nirlipta Tuli. Visit *yoganidranetwork.org/shop/sleep-well*

CBT-I. If you live in the UK, the NHS offers a service called Sleepstation that uses online learning in CBT-I (Cognitive Behavioural Therapy for Insomnia), including an app and individual coaching. Visit *thesleepclinic.org.uk*. For a similar program available in both the US and the UK, visit *sleepio.com*

Assessment of Sleep Issues. For assessment or advice on any sleep difficulty or issue, see the Sleep Unlimited services available at *sleepunlimited.co.uk*

Sleep School. Another program using CBT-I is the Sleep School's app, which has a daily Sleep Tracker Calendar, an Insomnia Survey, five audio tracks, and an interactive quiz. Visit *sleepschool.org*

Hypnotherapy. If you feel drawn to trying hypnotherapy, try the book and audio download *I Can Make You Sleep* by Paul McKenna (Bantam, 2009).

Apps, Gadgets, and Gear

Eye Pillows. It is claimed that eye pillows help relaxation by exerting gentle pressure on the eyelids, stimulating the vagus nerve. For more information, visit *yogaclicks.com/blogs/product-guides/the-gift-of-rest-eye-pillow-benefits-for-stress-and-sleep*

Stereo Headphones. Stereo headphones work best with audio files, and also reduce outside noise from traffic or snoring partners, particularly if they include a noise-cancelling option, but if they bother you, try using a single earpiece (search online for "mono earpiece with cup"), which you should find more comfortable. Or choose from the range of eyemasks that have built-in headphones. If you don't want the mask, go for "sleepphones", "pajamas for the ears". For more information, visit *sleepphones.com*

One company has now combined these kind of headband-style headphones with an app that offers you sleep-inducing stories and guided meditations. Visit Hoomband's website at *hoomsleep.com*

Weighted Blankets. Some people find their sleep improves using a weighted blanket that gives them a feeling of being secure and "hugged". Just search online for "weighted blanket".

Alarm Clock App. You can set alarms to both wake you up and remind you to go to bed in many smart phones now, but do not use sleep monitoring apps! (see page 24). If you want an alarm to wake you up at the optimal moment in your sleep cycle, the Sleep Cycle alarm clock app claims to wake you up in the lightest sleep phase. Visit *sleepcycle.com*

Blue-Light Blocking Glasses. If you just can't stop looking at those screens in the hour or so before bed, try wearing blue-light blocking glasses while you scroll and type (search for "blue-light blocking glasses").

Worry Diary. If you find you can't sleep because you worry when lying in bed, write down the worries in a journal, or "worry diary", to get them out of your head, or use the app from *worrywatch.com* (search in your app store for "Worry Watch: Anxiety Journal").

Sleep Story Podcasts and Apps. If you find listening to the human voice reading stories works for you, try the sleep story podcast *noth-ingmuchhappens.com*, or use the Sleep Stories section in the app from *calm.com*

Nature Sounds. Some people like the sound of rain outside, even a storm. There's an app that will provide you with many variations on this theme (search in your app store for "Infinite Storm").

Coloured Noise and Natural Sounds Machines. Machines that offer coloured noise and natural sounds are available from *soundof-sleep.com* and *soundofsleep.co.uk*

The Dodow Light Metronome. The Dodow is a machine that uses light and a metronome and claims to combine techniques from yoga, meditation, and behavioural therapy to train you to sleep better: For more information, visit *getdodow.io*

The Morphée. Try the Morphée, a beautifully designed aid to help you get to sleep using 210 variations of recordings in a male and female voice combining techniques from sophrology and mindfulness meditation, with a version, *My Little Morphée*, for children, too. Visit *morphee.co*

Low-Caffeine Coffees & Substitutes

In addition to the many coffee substitutes using ingredients like chicory, barley, or malt that have been around for decades, a new generation of no-caffeine or low-caffeine drinks is available, sometimes made with coffee and mushrooms, which include:

Four Sigmatic. *us.foursigmatic.com*

Mud\Wtr. *mudwtr.com*

Terpenes and CBD Cocktails. Information about terpenes and CBD cocktails can be found at *vogue.com/article/cannabis-terpene-cocktails-health-benefits*

Source of Terpenes. *Trueterpenes.com*

Snoring Fixes

If the quality of your sleep is being affected by your partner snoring, work through the potential sources of the problem: nose, mouth, or throat. And try the British Snoring & Sleep Apnoea Association's online test to find out what kind of snorer you are: *britishsnoring.co.uk/itests*

Nose. For the nose, try nose strips or Mute, a small device made of soft, adjustable material that sits inside your nose, increasing airflow and improving breathing: *mutesnoring.com*

Mouth. For the mouth, try a chin strap to hold your mouth closed or mouth tapes, available online.

Throat. For the throat, try special vocal exercises available from *singingforsnorers.com*. Or try a "snore mask", which analyzes the sound of your snoring and vibrates and allegedly makes the throat muscles tense, stopping you from snoring without even waking you up (search for "Beurer Snore Mask"). Or try a mandibular advancement device to hold the lower jaw and tongue forward, making more space to breathe and prevent snoring. For information, visit the British Snoring Association shop: *britishsnoring.co.uk*

The Sleep Foundation in the US reviews and recommends seven products on its website. Visit *sleepfoundation.org/best-anti-snoring-mouthpieces-and-mouthguards*

Smart Nora. A different route would be to allow the snoring but use a Smart Nora, a device that gently tips your head when you start snoring and will usually make you stop. For more information, visit *smartnora.com*

Sleeping Earplugs. If your sleep gets interrupted by external noise, such as traffic or your partner snoring, try sleeping earplugs, such as those available through *flareaudio.com/collections/sleeping*

Books

Antiglio, Dominique. *The Life-Changing Power of Sophrology: Breathe and Connect with the Calm and Happy You.* London: Yellow Kite/Hachette, 2018.

An exploration of sophrology that invites you to try it out and includes many anecdotes and real-life examples of its success.

Barrett, Deidre. *The Committee of Sleep: How Artists, Scientists, and Athletes Use Dreams for Creative Problem-Solving—and How You Can, Too.* New York: Crown/Random House, 2001.

How to work with the gift of the night to receive inspiration and solutions.

Carr-Gomm, Philip. *Empower Your Life with Sophrology: Quick and Simple Exercises to Reduce Stress, Boost Self-Esteem, and Help You Find Joy.* London: CICO Books, 2019.

A comprehensive introduction into the theory and practice of sophrology, with 26 accompanying audio-recordings, accessible here: *sophrology.institute/the-book*

De Carlo, Mar. *Awakening through Sleep: A Transformational and Spiritual Guide for Pregnancy, Adult, and Child Sleep.* The Baby Planner, 2020.

A starting point for exploring the topic for pregnant mothers and children's sleep.

Desai, Kamini. *Yoga Nidra: The Art of Transformational Sleep.* Twin Lakes, WI: Lotus Press, 2017.

An in-depth look at yoga nidra—how it works and the ways it can help you to relax, sleep, and meditate.

Dinsmore, Tuli, Uma & Nirlipta Tuli. *Yoga Nidra Made Easy: Deep Relaxation Practices to Improve Sleep, Relieve Stress, and Boost Energy and Creativity.* Carlsbad, CA: Hay House, 2022.

An inspiring and comprehensive survey by world experts on the topic.

His Holiness, the Dalai Lama, with Francisco J. Varela, Ph.D., ed. & narrator. *Sleeping, Dreaming, and Dying: An Exploration of Consciousness with the Dalai Lama.* Somerville, MA: Wisdom Publications, 2002.

In this account of a conference with the Dalai Lama and neuroscientists, these three states of consciousness and their relationships are explored from the perspectives of both the Tibetan Buddhist tradition and neuroscience.

Huffington, Arianna. *The Sleep Revolution: Transforming Your life One Night at a Time.* New York: Harmony, 2016.

A *New York Times* best-seller surveying our sleep-deprived culture, why we need better sleep, and some suggestions on how we can improve our sleep.

Hurd, Ryan. *Sleep Paralysis: A Guide to Hypnagogic Visions and Visitors of the Night.* Los Altos, CA: The Enlightened Hyena Press, 2020.

If parasomnias interest you, or if you are troubled with sleep paralysis, Ryan Hurd has researched this topic in depth.

Lee, David R. *Teaching the World to Sleep: Psychological and Behavioural Assessment and Treatment Strategies for People with Sleeping Problems and Insomnia.* New York: Routledge, 2018.

Although written for psychologists and health professionals, this comprehensive book will prove fascinating for the non-professional who is eager to go into the subject in depth.

Meadows, Guy, MD. *The Sleep Book: How to Sleep Well Every Night.* London: Orion, 2014.

A four-week program based on the author's experience treating insomnia using Cognitive Behavioural Therapy techniques and Mindfulness.

Naiman, Rubin, Ph.D. *Healing Night: The Science and Spirit of Sleeping, Dreaming, and Awakening.* CreateSpace, 2016.

Taking an integrative approach, Naiman combines information from contemporary medicine with a spiritual and Jungian perspective that encourages embracing darkness and the night as "sleep medicine".

Steiner, Rudoloph, with Michael Lipson, ed. & introduction. *Sleep and Dreams: A Bridge to the Spirit.* Hudson, NY: SteinerBooks, 2003.

In this collection of lectures, selected and introduced by the psychologist Michael Lipson, Steiner explores the idea that sleep, death, and meditation are the three realms in which consciousness has the opportunity to deepen its immersion in the divine flow of existence, with the aim of ultimately maintaining conscious awareness through all three states.

Stevenson, Shawn. *Sleep Smarter: 21 Essential Strategies to Sleep Your Way to a Better Body, Better Health, and Bigger Success.* Carlsbad, CA: Hay House, 2016.

Full of tips and information, this book also outlines a 14-day Sleep Makeover plan.

Stümpfig, Tina. *Jin Shin Healing Touch: Quick Help for Common Ailments.* Rochester, VT: Findhorn Press, 2020.

A step-by-step guide to the simple two-point touch method of Jin Shin Jyutsu for quick relief from many common conditions including sleeping problems.

Vernon, Alice. *Night Terrors: Troubled Sleep and the Stories We Tell About It.* London: Icon Books, 2022.

A lecturer in creative writing explores the way in which night terrors, sleep paralysis, and other parasomnias have influenced literature and story-telling.

Wiseman, Richard. *Night School: The Life-Changing Science of Sleep*. London: Pan Books 2015.
A witty and accessible review of sleep science, sufficiently full of anecdotes and fascinating facts to keep you awake even if reading in bed.

Walker, Matthew. *Why We Sleep: The New Science of Sleep and Dreams*. London: Penguin, 2017.
A best-seller that The London *Times* describes as "a powerful rallying cry by a researcher at the top of his game. If you want an effective distillation of a science that reaches deep into the frontiers of consciousness and identity . . . this is a good place to start."

Online Films

From two minutes' duration to an hour and a half, there are some great videos online about sleep: its benefits, its anomalies, the neuroscience of sleep, and how we can sleep better. Many of these are TED Talks. Use the eco-friendly search tool Ecosia to find them.

Online Training Courses

CBT-I. If you are a health or wellbeing professional and would like to learn how to deliver CBT-I, take a look at Dr. David Lee's Sleep Unlimited courses: *sleepunlimited.co.uk*

Holistic/Integrative Sleep Coach. If you are interested in training as a holistic/integrative sleep coach, visit *holisticsleepcoaching.com* and start with *sleep.com/adult-sleep-coach-certification*

Sophrology. If you'd like to train in sophrology, to help yourself and others, see my courses at The Sophrology Institute: *sophrology. institute/courses*

Sophrology/Silva Method. If you'd like a quick training in sophrology and the Silva Method, comparing and combining both, see the course on my website, Art of Living Well: *artoflivingwell.org.uk/p/ sophrologysilva*

Hypnotherapy. If you'd like to train in hypnotherapy, the specialist psychology training company Uncommon Knowledge offers a good online course: *unk.com*

Yoga Nidra. If you'd like to train in yoga nidra, see the online and in-person courses offered by the Yoga Nidra Network at *yoganidranetwork.org/teacher-training*

Lucid Dreaming. If you'd like to train in lucid dreaming, or are a therapist and want to learn how to incorporate lucid dream training into your work, see clinical psychologist Dr. Kristen LaMarca's programs at *mindfulluciddreaming.com*

Websites

The National Sleep Foundation. Created over 30 years ago in the US, the foundation offers a wide range of information on sleep, education, a journal, and awards. Its mission is to improve health and wellbeing through sleep education and advocacy: *thensf.org*

The Sleep Doctor. Clinical psychologist Dr. Michael Breus offers excellent information on sleep and how we can improve it. The website is full of articles that summarize every aspect of sleep and how we should best approach our sleep health: *thesleepdoctor.com*

Acknowledgements

I'd like to thank all those whose teaching, training, and advice helped me to develop the approach outlined in this book, and in particular Dorna Revie, who introduced me to the power of sophrology; Dr. Unsmore-Tuli and Nirlipta Tuli, who taught me how to teach yoga nidra; Dr. David Lee, whose CBT-I training was invaluable; Dr. Rosalind Watts, who introduced me to the world of psychedelic therapy; and Clare and Alexander Durdin Robertson, whose Huntington Castle and its gardens in Ireland provided me with the peace and inspiration to complete this book.

In addition, I'd like to thank all those who have taken my Sleep Clinic course and provided such helpful and encouraging feedback; my agent, Séverine Jeauneau; editorial director Sabine Weeke, editor Nicky Leach, and all the other good folks at Findhorn Press; and all those friends and colleagues whose editorial and other advice has contributed so much to this book.

About the Author

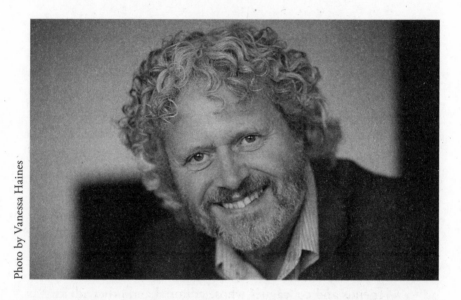

Photo by Vanessa Haines

Philip Carr-Gomm is an author and psychotherapist, trained in psychology, sophrology, and psychosynthesis psychotherapy. The founder of the Sophrology Institute, he works in the emerging field of psychedelic psychotherapy with the ACER Integration Community founded by Dr. Rosalind Watts.

Philip runs a sleep clinic that offers online sleep therapy and is the author of more than 20 books, including *Empower Your Life with Sophrology, Seek Teachings Everywhere,* and *The Prophecies*. He lives in Sussex, England.

For more information visit his website:
philipcarr-gomm.com

Index